Interventions for Disruptive Behaviors

The Guilford Practical Intervention in the Schools Series

Kenneth W. Merrell, Founding Editor
T. Chris Riley-Tillman, Series Editor

www.guilford.com/practical

This series presents the most reader-friendly resources available in key areas of evidence-based practice in school settings. Practitioners will find trustworthy guides on effective behavioral, mental health, and academic interventions, and assessment and measurement approaches. Covering all aspects of planning, implementing, and evaluating high-quality services for students, books in the series are carefully crafted for everyday utility. Features include ready-to-use reproducibles, lay-flat binding to facilitate photocopying, appealing visual elements, and an oversized format. Recent titles have Web pages where purchasers can download and print the reproducible materials.

Recent Volumes

Curriculum-Based Assessment for Instructional Design:
Using Data to Individualize Instruction
Matthew K. Burns and David C. Parker

Dropout Prevention
C. Lee Goss and Kristina J. Andren

Stress Management for Teachers: A Proactive Guide
Keith C. Herman and Wendy M. Reinke

Interventions for Reading Problems, Second Edition:
Designing and Evaluating Effective Strategies
*Edward J. Daly III, Sabina Neugebauer, Sandra Chafouleas,
and Christopher H. Skinner*

Classwide Positive Behavior Interventions and Supports:
A Guide to Proactive Classroom Management
Brandi Simonsen and Diane Myers

Promoting Academic Success with English Language Learners:
Best Practices for RTI
Craig A. Albers and Rebecca S. Martinez

The ABCs of CBM, Second Edition:
A Practical Guide to Curriculum-Based Measurement
Michelle K. Hosp, John L. Hosp, and Kenneth W. Howell

Integrated Multi-Tiered Systems of Support: Blending RTI and PBIS
Kent McIntosh and Steve Goodman

DBT Skills in Schools:
Skills Training for Emotional Problem Solving for Adolescents (DBT STEPS-A)
*James J. Mazza, Elizabeth T. Dexter-Mazza, Alec L. Miller, Jill H. Rathus,
and Heather E. Murphy*

Interventions for Disruptive Behaviors:
Reducing Problems and Building Skills
Gregory A. Fabiano

Promoting Student Happiness:
Positive Psychology Interventions in Schools
Shannon M. Suldo

Interventions for Disruptive Behaviors

Reducing Problems and Building Skills

GREGORY A. FABIANO

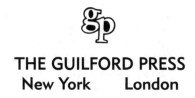

THE GUILFORD PRESS
New York   London

The author has checked with sources believed to be reliable in his efforts to provide information
that is complete and generally in accord with the standards of practice that are accepted at the
time of publication. However, in view of the possibility of human error or changes in behavioral,
mental health, or medical sciences, neither the author, nor the editor and publisher, nor any other
party who has been involved in the preparation or publication of this work warrants that the
information contained herein is in every respect accurate or complete, and they are not responsible
for any errors or omissions or the results obtained from the use of such information. Readers are
encouraged to confirm the information contained in this book with other sources.

Library of Congress Cataloging-in-Publication Data

Names: Fabiano, Gregory A., author.
Title: Interventions for disruptive behaviors : reducing problems and
    building skills / Gregory A. Fabiano.
Description: New York : The Guilford Press, 2016. | Series: The Guilford
    practical intervention in the schools series | Includes bibliographical
    references and index.
Identifiers: LCCN 2015045798| ISBN 9781462526611 (paperback) | ISBN
    9781462526703 (library pdf)
Subjects: LCSH: Behavior disorders in adolescence. | Behavior disorders in
    children. | Behavior therapy for children | Behavior therapy for
    teenagers. | BISAC: PSYCHOLOGY / Psychotherapy / Child & Adolescent. |
    MEDICAL / Psychiatry / Child & Adolescent. | SOCIAL SCIENCE / Social Work.
    | PSYCHOLOGY / Psychopathology / Attention-Deficit Disorder (ADD-ADHD).
Classification: LCC RJ506.B44 | DDC 618.92/89—dc23
LC record available at *https://lccn.loc.gov/2015045798*

*To my wife, Nora, who has taught me much
about the practical application of behavior management skills,
and to my children, Thomas, Julia, and Mary,
who are good sports and hard workers when we try out
behavior management approaches within our own family*

About the Author

Gregory A. Fabiano, PhD, is Professor of Counseling, School, and Educational Psychology in the Graduate School of Education at the University at Buffalo, State University of New York. He conducts research on evidence-based assessments and treatments for disruptive behavior disorders, with a particular focus on attention-deficit/hyperactivity disorder. Dr. Fabiano is a recipient of the Presidential Early Career Award for Scientists and Engineers, the nation's highest honor for early-career investigators. He is author or coauthor of over 70 peer-reviewed publications and book chapters.

Acknowledgments

This book is written to help parents, educators, and other professionals support youth with disruptive behavior disorders. I am indebted to the researchers and clinicians who have helped create, evaluate, and validate effective strategies for assessment and intervention directed to supporting youth with disruptive behavior disorders, as considerable prior work and effort informed the current text. In particular, William E. Pelham Jr. served as an outstanding mentor for me within graduate school (and beyond), providing multiple opportunities and excellent supervision, in order to foster the development of knowledge regarding best practices within school, home, and community settings.

I would also like to thank and acknowledge the many families, educators, and children with whom I have had the privilege to work, as together they provided the foundation of experiences that were drawn upon in writing this book.

Contents

CHAPTER 1

Introduction

In conceptualizing this book, I reflected on one of my earliest experiences as a child in elementary school, as well as on some recent experiences working with youth with disruptive behavior and their families. Looking back, I don't remember much about first grade, but I have a vivid memory of a hot June day at the end of the year. The teacher had said we could all go out for popsicles for recess before we went home on the bus. This was a real treat and out of the ordinary. The day seemed to crawl as we did our seatwork in a steaming hot classroom, and everyone looked forward to the special recess time. However, right before we were to go out, one of my classmates got upset at the teacher because he was asked to correct some errors on his seatwork. He got up from his chair, flipped over his desk, and started running around the room pulling papers off the wall. The teacher chased him, but the more she did, the more he ran around. Finally, a teacher from across the hall came over and the two adults marched the child down to the office. When the teacher came back, sweaty and disheveled from running around the room, she was so angry she said, "That's it! No popsicles today. We are all going to read quietly at our seats." This was one of my first experiences with disruptive behavior in the classroom, and I can state for certain that I did not enjoy the consequences of the behavior. This anecdote serves to demonstrate that the consequences of disruptive behavior go beyond the child exhibiting the behavior—the impact also reaches teachers, peers, and families, and therefore justifies intervention.

More recently, I spent some time working with a number of local districts to problem-solve behavior management. Although the districts were varied in terms of their neighborhoods, leadership, and the climate represented within the schools, it was remarkable how consistent the referring problems were to the child study teams. Teachers referred children who were not following rules, exhibiting disrespectful behavior toward adults and classmates, refusing to complete assigned work, and generally interfering with and interrupting classroom activities. The problems were frequent, ongoing, and stressful. Often the school staff lamented that the child's parents were not positively involved with the school. As the discussions on interventions progressed across the districts, it seemed like there were significant questions about the best approaches for dealing with the problems even though it was often remarked that the referred child had been sent to the committee across multiple school years. Notably, although many of the behaviors were challenging, I remained impressed with the professionalism and dedication of the educators who truly wanted the child to be successful and meet his or her potential within the classroom setting. Typically, I would also meet with the parents of referred children, and, not surprisingly, they too were searching for viable solutions, and they had been working to remediate the problem behaviors for a long time, often since preschool or earlier. Based on these experiences it seemed like it would be helpful to have a guidebook to assist in dealing with the challenges posed by disruptive behavior in positive and proactive ways for parents, educators, and others who support youth in our communities.

My interest in managing disruptive behavior has also increased given a shift I have seen in the field since I started working with youth with attention-deficit/hyperactivity disorder (ADHD) and associated disruptive behaviors in 1997. At that time, talking about medication for children with disruptive behavior was considered a taboo subject for educators, and parents were strongly opposed to the use of medication, only rarely using it as a "last resort." Sometime since then, things changed. I have heard children labeled as "untreated" if receiving no medication or when the parents decided to avoid "medical treatment" for the behavior. I have heard educators tell parents that they really should "go see the doctor" regarding the child's behavioral challenges. The emphasis on medication as part of intervention serves to outsource the partnership parents and educators should have in working together to promote school success for the child/teen. Although medication treatments are discussed here as part of a multimethod approach to intervention (see Chapter 8), one purpose of this book is to provide multiple approaches and strategies that should be attempted first, before medication is added as an adjunctive intervention on an as-needed basis.

Finally, contemporary approaches in the field have emphasized problem-solving frameworks in which tiered intervention approaches are commonly employed. Examples of such frameworks include positive behavioral interventions and supports (PBIS; Sugai et al., 1999) and response to intervention (RTI; Fletcher, Reid Lyon, Fuchs, & Barnes, 2007). These frameworks are useful to districts because they formalize the approach to intervention, and they include clear tiers of intervention intensity. However, educators and practitioners are often left wondering what interventions should be used within each of the levels of behavioral support, and at times they may have questions about how to best work with children across the levels. One goal of this book is to provide interveners with the tools necessary to realize the promise of these frameworks for preventing problems and supporting growth.

PURPOSE OF THIS BOOK

My intention in this book is to provide an overview of the identification, contextual influences, and interventions that are appropriate for youth with disruptive behaviors. Many sources exist to support these aims (e.g., DuPaul & Stoner, 2004; Lane, Menzies, Bruhn,

& Crnobori, 2010; Walker, Ramsey, & Gresham, 2003). This book serves to extend the literature by including resources, assessments, and strategies that may be useful for school practitioners across home, school, and community settings.

Within this book, when "disruptive behavior" is discussed, it serves as a catch-all for children who exhibit behaviors consistent with ADHD, oppositional defiant disorder (ODD), and conduct disorder (CD). Although children may exhibit ADHD, ODD, or CD individually, it is often the case that these disruptive behavior diagnoses are comorbid and co-occurring with one another. It also captures children classified as "other health impaired" (OHI) or "emotionally/behaviorally disturbed" (EBD) in school settings. Included under this descriptor are also children who exhibit challenging behaviors but do not meet criteria for mental health disorders or for special education classification. This is an important point to emphasize, as diagnoses in and of themselves do not result in referrals for intervention and treatment (Angold, Costello, Farmer, Burns, & Erkanli, 1999), diagnoses are unlikely to provide adequate prognostic information (e.g., Mannuzza & Klein, 1998), and diagnoses do not always describe the targeted behaviors that need to be addressed in intervention. Furthermore, the categorization itself does not represent the difficulties in daily functioning faced by the individual, or the needed areas for adaptive skills development. Indeed, simply knowing a diagnosis or categorization does not provide any information on the context within which the problem behavior occurs, something that is critical to know about if effective interventions are to be implemented. Thus, throughout the book a functional approach to assessment and intervention will be adopted (see Chapter 2).

OVERVIEW OF THE CONTEXT FOR TREATING DISRUPTIVE BEHAVIOR

When children misbehave and exhibit disruptive, oppositional, or rule-breaking behavior, the typical approach within our society is to reprimand, punish, or scold. If there is any doubt about this, one simply has to go to a local grocery store or classroom and observe how adults interact with youth. You will readily observe adults saying things like "Don't run!"; "Stop that!"; and "You're getting on my nerves!" Children who are following rules, complying with commands, and exhibiting respectful behavior rarely have similar amounts of attention directed toward them when these appropriate behaviors occur, and the already low levels recede even further as children progress from the primary grades to middle and high school. Indeed, because negative and disruptive behaviors are externalizing and therefore very easy to observe, they often become one of the main targets of adult attention.

The consequences of this approach to dealing with disruptive behavior are perhaps best illustrated via anecdote. I will describe two children. The first child is my son. By all accounts, he developed typically. Even at 2 months old his day care teachers told us he was a good baby and easy to feed and get to nap. At preschool, my wife and I were very proud of the pictures he drew, and we posted them on our refrigerator. We enjoyed talking with him about his day and learning about what he had for snack and who he played with during free time. When he went to kindergarten, we were proud to see him get on the bus on his own, and also proud to hear positive reports from his teacher about his behavior and his progress in school. Then he went to first grade. During the first week of school, I received a panicked call from my wife that we had received a note from the teacher stating that our son was talking during quiet time. Of course, the two of us were beside ourselves with this negative news! As I drove home from work that day, I was trying to decide how to handle it. When I got home, I told my wife I was not sure what to do, and she looked at me incredulously and said, "But you're the child psychologist!" I looked back and said, "But you're his mother. You always know what to do!" Eventually, we decided we were going to make him write a note to the teacher apologizing for his behavior. As one might imagine, for a beginning first grader, a writing assignment can be very unpleasant because the ability to write is not yet fluid. It took our son almost 40 minutes to complete the note, and the process involved lots of tears. However, eventually he finished the note and we told him he needed to hand it to his teacher and apologize the next day.

The next day was a long one for my wife and me. We were both anxiously waiting for our son to get off the bus so we could find out how his day went. I think we were both nervous that there would be more trouble at school, and we strongly wanted our son to return to his typical good behavior in the classroom. I got a call from my wife at 2:30 when my son came home on the bus, and I got the news. She said, "I asked him how the day went and he said good. When I asked him about the note he told me the teacher said she was surprised he wrote it because it wasn't that big of a deal." Well it was a big deal for us!

Our son is now in sixth grade, and although he is certainly not perfect, for the most part he has gone through the rest of school without much in the way of additional negative feedback. There has been an occasion or two where he has gotten in trouble or made a bad choice, but we have been able to deal with these situations and correct them. Overall, across his whole school career, we have had three instances of negative feedback about his behavior relative to multiple positive and supportive comments, report cards, and teacher notes. His school career to this point is representative of most children within school settings with regard to feedback—the majority experience no or neutral feedback with a little positive feedback sprinkled in, and negative feedback almost never happens.

So, I have told you about one child, with what I think is a fairly typical school experience—a few situations where corrective feedback is necessary are embedded within an overall positively valanced environment. Now let's consider a child with the disruptive behavior disorders I will be focusing on within this book. Furthermore, rather than focusing on a whole school career from early day care until sixth grade, let's focus on a single day for an 8-year-old-child with disruptive behavior challenges.

The day is likely to begin with a parent coming into the room to wake up the child (7:00 A.M.). Because school is often an unsuccessful place to be, there is little motivation on the part of the child to go to school, so the response to the parent's "Rise and shine" comment is to pull the covers over his head. Thus, the day begins with a parent request (admittedly a vague one) met with noncompliance. After some additional prompts that go unheeded, the parent may eventually rip the covers off and sternly tell the child to get up and get dressed

(7:05 A.M.). As the parent leaves to begin to get herself ready for the day, the child busies himself with a half-made Lego set. When the parent comes back to see the child still in his pajamas, a more irritated set of commands to get ready for school will result (7:10 A.M.). As the child begins to get dressed, he may do so in a disorganized fashion or slowly, resulting in more parental commands to get dressed appropriately (7:10–7:20 A.M.). Because the child did not put his shoes in the front hall the night before, considerable time is spent looking for the shoes, which are eventually found in an unusual place for shoes: under the couch. The search for shoes includes a long lecture from the parent regarding the need to put things back where they belong because this happens all the time (7:20–7:25 A.M.). Once dressed, the child sits down for breakfast and because he is reaching to grab a magazine his sister is reading, he spills a full glass of orange juice all over the table and gets his parent's coat on the chair soaked and sticky. His parent, now angry, yells at him to get his backpack and head outside toward the bus stop (7:30 A.M.). On the way to the bus stop at the corner, the parent scolds the child to "not bother the other kids like yesterday and just stand still!" The child, excited to see the other kids, gets upset when they do not reciprocate his excitement, and teases one in front of the other parents, resulting in a reprimand from his own parent and a number of cold stares from the other children's parents. Finally, the bus arrives and the child's exasperated parent says, "Finally, the bus is here" and briskly walks back to the home without looking back (7:35 A.M.).

This might be considered a negative morning, but it does not stop here. As the children file onto the bus, the bus driver stops the child and says, "Listen, I have had enough of your fooling around and moving from seat to seat. From now on you have an assigned seat right behind me in the front row." Because this is typically where kindergarten children sit, the other children laugh at and tease the child from the back rows (7:35–7:50 A.M.). As the child exits the bus, he gets stared down by the bus monitor, who had previously been welcoming every prior child to school by name, but who now says, "You better walk!" before he even gets off the bus and has a chance to make the choice to walk or run (7:50 A.M.).

Then the child enters the classroom and instead of hanging up his coat and putting his backpack in his cubby like the other children, he walks back to the corner of the classroom where the class turtle is located to look at it and see how it is doing. As he is distracted by the turtle, his classmates are sitting down and beginning their bellwork (7:50–8:00 A.M.). When the teacher notices him in the back of the room, the first thing she says to him is "Why aren't you ready? I hope today is not going to be another one of your days like yesterday because I am not in the mood to deal with it!" (8:00 A.M.).

To recap, within the first hour of the day this child has had more negative interactions with parents, siblings, peers, teachers, and other adults than most typically developing kids have within their entire school careers! Until this context is acknowledged, identified, and changed, forward progress is unlikely to occur. It is no wonder that when we plan interventions for youth with disruptive behavior that they do not work right away, or even after a few weeks. Indeed, it is foolish to think a couple of stickers on a chart or a one-time reward will reasonably improve behavior when this is offered within the context of a pervasively and chronically negative environment. Within this context, punishments are also unlikely to work because the child's whole environment is already punishing. Doling out punishments within an already negative context is like putting water on a grease fire: they are likely to only make the situation worse and more difficult to control. Notably, there are also different functional explanations for the child and adult behaviors (see Chapter 2), making a one-size-fits-all approach unlikely to be effective. This example of a prototypical child with challenging behavior underscores the need for coordinated, sustained, positively focused interventions for youth with disruptive behavior disorders.

BRIEF REVIEW OF A THEORETICAL MODEL OF CREATING AND SUSTAINING DISRUPTIVE BEHAVIOR

Gerald Patterson (1982) was an early pioneer of the study of the nature, causes, and interventions for youth with disruptive behavior disorders. One of his key contributions to the field was a theoretical framework that used social learning theory as a way to explain the development of disruptive behavior disorders within the family context. He called this pattern a "coercive family process" and defined it as a process through which negative child behaviors and parental attention administered through reprimands or correction occur reciprocally within a cycle of reinforcement, strengthening maladaptive patterns over time. Thus, the negative behaviors escalate due to an attempt to override parental consequences (e.g., punishments).

The coercive family process is best described through an example. Let's think about a young child who does not want to eat her vegetables. During dinnertime, she might initially whine when offered vegetables and avoid eating them. Her mother may command or coax her into eating her vegetables, but after some time might give up this effort. Thus, the child is negatively reinforced because the demand to eat a food she dislikes is removed. Importantly, the mother is also negatively reinforced because she no longer has to deal with irritating child behavior. However, the next time the mother attempts to place the demand of eating vegetables on the child, it happens within the context of this historical event where the child was successful in having the demand removed following the whining behavior. This next time, she may not only complain but physically push the plate away when her mother instructs her to eat her vegetables. The mother may now raise her voice and repeat the commands, but if she relents, the child has now learned that increasing her negative behavior may be a useful tool for influencing her mother's behavior. If we fast forward across many dinners and many requests to eat her vegetables, it is not necessarily hard to envision how the situation could eventually involve the mother screaming at her child and the child throwing vegetables at the mother. This very serious situation that includes harsh parenting and extremely negative child behavior is the culmination of a number of insidious, transactional parent–child interactions that over time escalate and strengthen the negative behavior exhibited by the child and the maladaptive approach to parenting this child in this situation. The framework of this theoretical model of coercive family process provides natural areas to target within effective intervention approaches, as described below.

EVIDENCE-BASED TREATMENTS FOR DISRUPTIVE BEHAVIOR DISORDERS

Fortunately for individuals who work to support youth with disruptive behavior disorders, there is a strong evidence base of interventions with which to work. The best interventions for youth with disruptive behavior in general, those with ADHD, and those with ODD/CD will be reviewed, followed by a discussion of best practice approaches to intervention.

Treatments for Disruptive Behaviors

To some degree it is "funny" to try to make an argument that evidence-based treatments should be used for disruptive behavior disorders. After all, who would take the position that one should use "non-evidence-based practices"? Yet, many of the treatments used for disruptive behavior disorders are not supported by evidence, including individual counseling, school grade retentions, suspensions, and expulsions, and "shock" interventions such as taking the child to a police station or prison to "scare the child straight."

Although it may seem obvious, the emphasis on using evidence-supported treatments that have been vetted within controlled research has only been present in the field for a relatively short period of time. In the late 1980s and the early 1990s the medical field began to identify and recommend that doctors use approaches supported by research evidence. This movement served as a model for psychology and education, where child treatments for disruptive behavior disorders have been formally evaluated and the approaches with supporting evidence have been identified (e.g., Brestan & Eyberg, 1998; Pelham, Wheeler, & Chronis, 1998; also see the website *http://ies.ed.gov/ncee/wwc*). Currently, there are professional treatment guidelines for pediatricians and psychiatrists, teachers, and consumers that provide reviews of the state of the evidence for treatments used to support youth with disruptive behavior disorders.

Thus it is important to explicitly state that the position of this book is that the treatments employed for youth with disruptive behavior disorders should be based on research evidence that indicates effectiveness for the approach. Although it is difficult to state equivocally that a particular intervention is evidence-based as new evidence can be continually accruing, in a situation where there is evidence in support of a particular intervention, this will be the chosen emphasis in treatment planning relative to an intervention without supportive evidence.

Resources are available for managing disruptive behaviors using evidence-based practices in homes and schools. A nice guide for educators was disseminated by the U.S. Department of Education that describes best-practice foundational strategies for use in schools (Epstein, Atkins, Cullinan, Kutash, & Weaver, 2008). This practice guide suggests a clear, stepwise approach to behavior management grounded in a large literature. The first step includes conducting a good functional analysis of the targeted behavior. Next, the educator should modify the classroom environment to promote positive behaviors (i.e., antecedent control; see Chapter 5). Next, the teacher teaches and reinforces new skills and appropriate behaviors (see Chapter 6). Following this, educators adopt schoolwide strategies, as needed (see Chapter 10).

Similar findings have been recommended for young children. Hemmeter, Fox, Jack, and Broyles (2007) describe a positive behavioral support model appropriate for early childhood settings. In this approach, foundational strategies that include building strong relationships with children and families are emphasized for the whole class. This includes simply ensuring there are more positive than negative interactions with children and parents. Furthermore, as in the Epstein and colleagues (2008) practice guide for elementary schools, environmental modifications are made to ensure appropriate behavior is maximized in the classroom. In addition, educators are supported in their teaching of social and emotional skills, something that may be particularly relevant for young children who are becoming socialized to a structured school setting. Finally, any children that still require support and intervention receive individualized positive behavioral support strategies on an ongoing basis.

Treatments for ADHD

An additional line of research has identified effective interventions for youth with ADHD. ADHD is a disruptive behavior disorder characterized by developmentally inappropriate levels of inattention, hyperactivity, and impulsivity. These behaviors are pervasive, meaning they occur across settings. Furthermore, they are long-standing, meaning that they occur over long periods of time, across development; current conceptualizations of ADHD consider it to be a life-course-persistent disorder that begins in childhood and continues through adolescence into adulthood (American Academy of Pediatrics, 2011). Finally, and perhaps most importantly, ADHD results in considerable impairment in daily life functioning across major life domains including peer relationships, adult interactions and relationships, academic progress and functioning, family functioning, and work situations (American Psychiatric Association, 2013; Fabiano et al., 2006).

Multiple treatments have been tried to reduce ADHD behaviors and problems. Among the most common interventions are the stimulant medications (e.g., Ritalin, Adderall, Dexedrine, Concerta, Focalin). A discussion of this intervention is elaborated in Chapter 8. A broader category of potential intervention includes psychological or psychosocial treatment. This might include one-to-one counseling, family therapy, parent training programs, token economies or other behavior management programs, social skills training, cognitive-behavioral therapy, exercise programs, neurofeedback, cognitive training programs (i.e., working memory training), and other treatments such as withholding potential allergens, food dyes, and sugars, or by providing supplements such as vitamins or natural extracts.

Out of all of these interventions, the number without an evidence base dwarfs the number with an evidence base. There is no evidence that one-on-one counseling provides an effective remediation of ADHD symptoms or impairment. This makes sense if one really thinks about it—youth with ADHD often do not have challenges within one-on-one situations. Problems are much more likely to occur in group settings such as families, classrooms, or sports teams when the child experiences behavioral demands. Furthermore, youth with

ADHD often have poor insight into their own problems, overestimating their contributions to success in their functioning and underestimating their role in failures in functioning (Owens et al., 2007). This attributional style does not align well with insight-oriented therapies or counseling approaches that require the individual to account for his or her own role in his or her current difficulties. Coupled with the young age of many children with ADHD, this approach, although commonly recommended and employed, is not an effective way to help. There are also numerous other treatments that have been debunked or not critically evaluated for ADHD. These include biofeedback, play therapy, cognitive training, and individual social skills training. These treatments are limited because they also occur outside the typical situations where youth with ADHD have difficulties. There is little evidence within the field that children with ADHD can effectively generalize any strategies presented within a one-to-one treatment to a novel situation. Furthermore, although many parents are adamant that food dyes, sugars, or other foods *cause* ADHD behavior, controlled trials have repeatedly illustrated that these substances do not have an appreciable effect on the behavior of youth with ADHD (Wolraich, Wilson, & White, 1995), except perhaps in individuals with known food sensitivities.

So, what does work in the treatment of ADHD? There is consensus that three approaches meet predetermined criteria for calling an intervention "evidence-based." Multiple reviews (Fabiano, Schatz, Aloe, Chacko, & Chronis-Tuscano, 2015; Pelham et al., 1998; Pelham & Fabiano, 2008) including different review teams (Evans, Owens, & Bunford, 2013) have concluded that three interventions have acceptable empirical support from well-designed research studies as treatments that work for ADHD. These three interventions are behavioral parent training (see Chapter 4), contingency management procedures employed by teachers in schools (see Chapter 5), and training interventions that teach the child or teen specific, adaptive skills (see Chapter 6). Because they are evidence-based interventions and therefore the best approach for an effective treatment plan for individuals with ADHD, there is a specific chapter dedicated to each.

Treatments for ODD and CD

There are also evidence-based approaches for ODD and CD. Notably, the comorbidity between youth with ADHD and ODD/CD is high, so in many cases treatment providers, parents, and educators are likely to be dealing with behaviors representative of multiple categorical disorders. Reviews of best-practice interventions for children with ODD and CD yield similar conclusions to the reviews for ADHD treatment, at least with respect to psychosocial treatments. Systematic reviews clearly support behavioral parent training as an evidence-based intervention for youth with ODD/CD (Eyberg, Nelson, & Boggs, 2008). Eyberg and colleagues (2008) review over a dozen parent training interventions for ODD/CD and conclude that most meet criteria as probably efficacious treatments for these disruptive behavior disorders. The main reason for most of the parent training programs failing to be classified in the strongest evidence category (well established) is that there were not multiple clinical trials conducted by independent investigatory teams for each specific parent training "package." However, if the literature is viewed through a different lens, and the treatment is conceptualized as simply "parent training," there are now dozens of studies that document positive results for youth with disruptive behavior following parent training. Thus, like treatment studies for ADHD, there is clear evidence supporting behavioral parent training for youth with ODD/CD.

SUMMARY AND OVERVIEW OF THE BOOK

Following this chapter is a description of the approach to conceptualizing disruptive behaviors that uses a functional rather than a psychiatric diagnostic approach (Chapter 2). Chapter 3 reviews assessment strategies that are appropriate for different purposes that might be clinical goals when working with youth with disruptive behaviors and their families. There are a number of foundational strategies that are effective for youth with challenging behaviors. Chapter 4 outlines these strategies that may be used by parents, and Chapter 5 outlines these strategies for educators. In Chapter 6, approaches for teaching adaptive skills are reviewed. Chapter 7 reviews approaches to training interventions that are useful for promoting the development and use of adaptive skills. Chapter 8 deals with medications commonly used to treat disruptive behavior disorders. Chapter 9 discusses common strategies for employing integrated and engaging interventions for family units over long periods of time, an approach that is likely to be needed for the majority of youth experiencing problems in functioning due to disruptive behavior. Finally, Chapter 10 provides an overview of how the strategies reviewed in this book might be deployed within school systems in a problem-solving framework.

CHAPTER 2

A Function-Based Approach to Intervention

CATEGORIZATION

The world is filled with categories and labels. A person works in a white-collar or a blue-collar profession. We drive a compact car or an SUV. Fast-food restaurants serve breakfast or lunch, depending on the time of day. She lives in the United States or in Canada. These categories are helpful, as they help people rapidly sort information in a generally efficient way. However, this efficiency can have a cost at times in that broad categorization ignores individual differences that do not fit neatly into any particular category.

In schools, categories are often used as well. There are kindergarteners, first graders, and 10th graders. Children are elementary schoolers, middle schoolers, or high schoolers. Children may also be in general education or special education. Within special education, there may be a number of additional categories such as other health impaired (OHI), speech–language impaired (SLI), and emotionally–behaviorally disturbed (EBD); some children meet criteria for multiple categories and are therefore placed in another category called "multiply disabled." One of the most important categories within schools is graduated versus not graduated. These categories are again useful as they permit children to be efficiently grouped into classrooms, programs, and policies, and others within the school system can make rapid generalizations about the child based on the categorical distinctions. For instance, it would be helpful for a school counselor to know ahead of time whether he or she is meeting with a kindergartener or a 12th grader for a session, as the preparation would be quite different, depending on the child's grade.

Disruptive behavior disorders have also been subjected to categorization strategies. The *Diagnostic and Statistical Manual of Mental Disorders* (5th ed. [DSM-5]; American Psychiatric Association, 2013) includes multiple categorical diagnoses for disruptive behavior disorders. In the DSM-5, diagnoses are dichotomously classified: they are either present or not present. Children and adolescents are required to have a predetermined number of symptoms endorsed as present, the symptoms need to cause psychosocial impairment, and a clinician needs to rule out other explanations for the presentation of symptoms (e.g., a medical cause). Most diagnoses are established through interviews with parents and teachers to ascertain information on the presence of symptoms as well as their impact on daily life functioning. This categorical diagnostic approach has predominated in the field of child psychology and mental health for the past 40 years.

In parallel, many school systems have also embraced a categorical approach for special education placement and services. Traditionally, children with behavioral concerns would be referred for an evaluation to determine whether special education services were warranted. This assessment approach typically involved a series of assessments (e.g., cognitive, achievement), teacher and parent interviews and rating scales, and classroom observations that aimed to identify whether a student was in need of special education services, supports, and/or placements, due to a disability in a functional domain that impaired his or her ability to learn. This categorical approach had been widely employed in school settings for decades.

CONCERNS ABOUT THE CATEGORICAL APPROACH

In spite of widespread use, recent research studies, public policy decisions, and the experiences of children and families have raised concerns about this categorical approach to the provision of mental health and school services. For one, categorical approaches are a stark approach to description with little room for the complexities and originalities within children. This is illustrated by a traditional approach to the placement of children in special education services for reading wherein a significant discrepancy between estimated IQ and academic achievement was required. In these instances, a committee on special education might require greater than a 20-point difference between the child's assessment of cognitive ability (i.e., IQ) and his or her academic achievement (i.e., in reading or math). Thus, a child with an IQ of 100 and a reading achievement score of 79 would be eligible for special education supports and placements, but a child with a comparable IQ and an achievement score of 80 would not be eligible, even though this might practically mean a difference of only one to two words read on the assessment. This categorical approach would also present some difficulties in other cases—a child with an IQ of 130 with average achievement scores in reading (e.g., 100) would have a large discrepancy, but would be functioning at expected achievement levels. Using a categorical approach this child would be eligible for services whereas one with low achievement scores (i.e., 70) at a comparable level of cognitive ability (i.e., IQ = 82) would not qualify. However, one might logically argue that the child in the second case would also warrant supportive interventions to attain grade-level competencies.

By way of another example, consider a child brought to the pediatrician's office due to behavioral concerns who has a parent and teacher endorse five symptoms of ADHD rather than six. This child does not meet diagnostic criteria, but may still have behavioral challenges that warrant treatment. If this child is experiencing peer impairments such as rejection, bullying, or socialization struggles; failing to complete expected tasks in the classroom; and disrupting group activities in the classroom and on sports teams, it would be foolish to tell the family that their child does not warrant intervention because he or she did not surpass a threshold of a requisite number of symptoms that is arbitrarily constructed (i.e., there is little evidence that six symptoms are clinically meaningful or important relative to other potential cutoffs or combinations of symptoms; Pelham, Fabiano, & Massetti, 2005). Most would agree that this child warrants intervention regardless of whether diagnostic thresholds are surpassed, given the evidence of impairment in functioning. This example is supported by research that shows impairment in functioning is what predicts treatment seeking more strongly than the presence of symptoms related to diagnosis (Angold et al., 1999).

An additional problem with the categorical approach is that the categories can become "shortcuts" for practitioners that then lead to one-size-fits-all treatment that may or may not be helpful to the targeted child. For instance, consider the heuristic "If a child is diagnosed with ADHD, he should get stimulant medication"; this is a shortcut that can have a number of negative implications such as ignoring parent/child preference for treatment, reducing the realm of treatment options that might be helpful, and marginalizing the importance of school supports. Sometimes the categorical diagnosis works in an opposite direction. There was once a local residential treatment facility that would not accept children with CD because of concerns regarding aggressive behavior. Some providers became loathe to provide this diagnosis for children due to a concern of limiting their range of potential referral sources for treatment, so the diagnostic approach shifted to categorizing all these youth as ODD instead.

Perhaps one of the most relevant contemporary examples is the dramatic increase in pediatric bipolar diagnoses. The diagnosis of bipolar disorder has been well established for over a century in adults, and it is characterized by "a distinct period of abnormally and persistently elevated, expansive, or irritable mood and abnormally and persistently increased goal-directed activity or energy, lasting at least one week and present most of the day, nearly every day" (American Psychiatric Association, 2013, p. 124). Furthermore, to be diagnosed with bipolar disorder, "The mood disturbance is sufficiently severe to cause marked impairment in social or occupational functioning or to necessitate hospitalization to prevent harm to self or others, or there are psychotic features" (American Psychiatric Association, 2013, p. 124). This is describing severe mental illness, and anyone who has been around an individual who is in a manic or major depressive episode is likely to describe the individual as very impaired and to determine that the individual needs intensive psychiatric intervention such as hospitalization. In contrast, beginning in the 2000s many practitioners began ascribing a "pediatric bipolar" diagnosis to youth who were irritable, frustrated easily, distractible, behaved impulsively, talked excessively, and had difficulty settling down at night to go to sleep. Unfortunately, these behaviors overlap with ADHD/ODD/CD symptoms as well. Thus, it is often unclear whether these behaviors represent a distinct mood state or are better conceptualized as part of a developmental, disruptive behavior disorder. Unfortunately, depending on the label used to ascribe the behaviors, quite different treatments may result. Considering just medication, a child with ADHD may be prescribed a stimulant; a child with ODD/CD may be prescribed nothing at all or a medication intended to reduce aggression but prescribed in a fashion not approved by the U.S. Food and Drug Administration (FDA), such as an atypical antipsychotic; and a child diagnosed with pediatric bipolar disorder may be prescribed lithium or another mood-regulating drug. Here the labels are being used as heuristics and shortcuts for treatment, while a good functional assessment of the behaviors, environmental contributors, and variables maintaining the behaviors is missing.

A final problem with a categorical approach to diagnosis is that the diagnosis or classifications in and of themselves do not provide prescriptive information on the specific intervention or combinations of interventions that will work. Furthermore, educational classifications such as "OHI" or "CD" do not provide the needed descriptive information on the behaviors that contribute to the classification presently and in the past, the functions of the behaviors, or the other contextual features that might contribute to the case conceptualization and eventual treatment plan. A child classified as CD could be extremely aggressive, extremely covert and sneaky with respect to negative behaviors (e.g., lying or stealing), engaging in serious rule violations (e.g., skipping school, running away), or some combination of all these behaviors. The label thus provides very little actionable information for educators and treatment providers overall.

Some of the limitations of a categorical approach to diagnosis have been provided. This discussion would be remiss if some of the reasons the categorical approach has taken hold were not also reviewed. The categorical approach is favored by insurance companies looking to establish a diagnosis that would warrant treatment, diagnoses are also useful within research settings for appropriately classifying the participants within the study, and school districts may use categorical labels as a means of "gatekeeping" for the appropriate use of services and accommodations. It should also be emphasized that the diagnostic process, including a summative diagnosis, may be of comfort for parents who are dealing with disruptive behaviors as it provides a label to justify the stress and challenges the family has experienced. However, beyond these reasons, it is difficult to think of additional ways categorical labels enhance the treatment enterprise. As diagnostic assessments within child psychology and educational settings should be thought of as formative rather than summative, the categorical (summative) approach is a serious limitation of current diagnostic approaches. Given this reality, there are some approaches advocated and utilized within the field that can be used as a launching point for the assessments described within Chapter 3.

ADVANTAGES OF A FUNCTIONAL APPROACH

A framework for conceptualizing assessment and intervention that uses a function-based approach can potentially offer a number of advantages. These are nicely described by Scotti, Morris, McNeil, and Hawkins (1996), who outline some of the same limitations of the categorical diagnoses described above, and who suggest that functional assessments of behaviors may be an approach with more merit and utility. Considering disruptive behavior disorders, even if a child has a diagnosis of ODD with specific symptoms endorsed (e.g., is often angry and resentful, often defies or refuses to comply with an adult's requests or rules, deliberately annoys others), a clinician is still left with little actionable information. There is no information within the data collected for a diagnosis that informs the clinician on setting events, the individuals with whom these behaviors occur or they are directed toward, potential antecedents of the problem behavior, consequences that follow the behaviors, potential antecedents and consequences that might attenuate the problem behaviors or maintain them, competencies that might need to be built for the child and family by the clinician, and areas of strength that are present. Thus, a clinician could spend considerable time on the diagnostic process and still be left at the end needing to spend an additional considerable amount of time to inform treatment planning. Furthermore, whether these diagnoses are alone or comorbid tells a clinician little to nothing about what intervention would be the correct approach. Educators could come to the same conclusion if they are told a student is OHI, EBD, or learning disabled (LD); these categorical labels lack the clinically meaningful information needed to support and appropriately educate the student using differentiated instruction strategies, tailor behavioral interventions in a manner that supports the child's behavior and learning, and foster the appropriate environment for growth in social and academic functioning.

An example of this includes an RTI approach. Although this approach includes categorical groupings within its framework, the goal of RTI is to extend the range of categories from a dichotomous system (i.e., general education or special education) to a system that includes more groupings (i.e., Tiers 1, 2, and 3). Furthermore, Tiers 1 and 2 precede Tier 3, typically the tier consistent with special education. Thus, schools are currently moving away from a dichotomous approach to categorization toward an approach with more attention toward levels of intervention that are administered dependent on need (e.g., Fletcher et al., 2007).

At a federal level there has also been increased emphasis on continuous, dimensional descriptions of behavior that rise above traditional categorical distinctions. The National Institutes of Mental Health (2014) recently pioneered "Research Domain Criteria" (RDoC). The RDoC criteria were created as an alternative to the traditional DSM classification approach. They classify mental health disorders on a continuum of behavioral dimensions and integrate neurobiological measures as well. The RDoC approach begins with the study of basic processes such as how a child processes social information, how rewards influence behavior, or how memories are stored and manipulated. Integrated into these basic research questions are the influences of genetics and underlying biological processes such as neurotransmitter activity and brain function, including how these may influence observable behaviors. Taken together, these basic research studies provide information on underlying mechanisms that may result in observed problems or adaptive behaviors. Then, these mechanisms can be studied across traditional diagnostic categories, resulting in study samples that are more homogeneous and therefore better able to answer precise questions about developmental psychopathology, treatment development and response, and prevention efforts.

This approach to classification as a formative assessment of targeted behaviors is not new. A perusal of the initial issues of the *Journal of Applied Behavior Analysis*, which included many interventions used with youth with disruptive behavior disorders, reveals few diagnoses but rather comprehensive descriptions of the nature, frequency, and type of referring problems. This is exemplified by Patterson's pioneering work. In his early studies of behavioral parent training for youth with disruptive behaviors, he did not have a DSM manual, lengthy structured interviews to determine diagnoses, multiday evaluations by school psychologists, or neuropsychological batteries to determine whether they were experiencing behavior problems. He simply treated target behaviors, also known as the reason the parent sought out treatment in the first place. In one of his early publications (Patterson, 1975a), families were referred for treatment because of "high rates of aggressive behavior" (p. 304). The report includes a table describing these referring problems, ranging from "lies, fights with sibs, steals, tantrums, argues" to "temper tantrums, not minding, wets bed, soils" to "fights, noncomply, hyperactive, noisy" to "fights, noncomply, hyperactive, argues, nausea, insomnia, giddiness (Patterson, 1975a, p. 315). Represented within these symptoms are potential characteristics of ADHD, ODD, CD, enuresis, encopresis, and perhaps even mood disorder. Yet, it was not necessary for a structured interview and DSM diagnosis to be conducted in order to effectively treat these youth. These clinically rich descriptions clearly and explicitly identify target behaviors that are then addressed in treatment. Importantly, the functional assessment is unitary with treatment planning—that is, in the process of defining behaviors that justify intervention the clinician or educator is also identifying targets of intervention. By way of one other example, Witt and Elliott (1982) effectively improved the behavior of three children selected because the teacher said "they were the most severe behavior problems in the class." Although there is no other information on the specific behaviors that resulted in the teacher's concern, clearly the children's behaviors resulted in school impairment (there is a comment that each child had been suspended on at least one occasion), and the treatment efforts utilized within the classroom were warranted. Because the intervention focused on a socially valid targeted outcome—classroom rule violations—specific diagnoses for the youth were not needed.

FUNCTION-BASED ASSESSMENTS: AN ALTERNATIVE APPROACH

A number of limitations to a dichotomous approach to classification have been outlined. As is discussed further (see Chapter 3), a functional approach to assessment is recommended. This is an assessment that attempts to determine *why* a problem behavior is occurring (its function) and *what* is maintaining it (its antecedents and consequences). Basically, a functional assessment uncovers the possible reason why a behavior that is problematic continues to be exhibited by the child: there must be some reason the behavior makes sense from the child's perspective or else it would not be exhibited in the first place and on a continuing basis. To use an obvious example, think of a child who dislikes completing math worksheets. During math time this child stands up, throws his entire desk over, and is promptly sent to the principal's office. Math worksheets are something most children dislike, but for some children this task is so strongly disliked that the child may go to great lengths to avoid them, even if it means other consequences may occur. It makes sense to exhibit the disruptive behavior of turning over the desk as it affords the child the opportunity to *avoid* completing the math work. If the child's goal is to avoid/escape the task of completing math worksheets, this disruptive behavior is highly effective for doing so! Longer-term consequences such as getting into trouble with the principal or at home may not make as much sense to this particular child as the immediate avoidance of a disliked task.

Now let's return to the example in Chapter 1 of the child with disruptive behavior challenges beginning his school day. Throughout the vignette, the possible functional reasons for the negative behaviors are listed in **bold** in the parentheses:

> The day is likely to begin with a parent coming into the room to wake up the child (7:00 A.M.). Because school is often an unsuccessful place, there is no motivation on the part of the child to go to school so the response to the parent's "Rise and shine" comment is to pull the covers over his head (**avoidance**). Thus, the day begins with a parent request (admittedly a vague one) met with noncompliance. After some additional prompts that go unheeded, the parent may eventually rip the covers off and sternly tell the child to get up and get dressed (7:05 A.M.). As the parent leaves to begin to get herself ready for the day, the child busies himself with a half-made Lego set (**avoidance—getting dressed is a tedious activity**). When the parent comes back to see the child still in his pajamas, a more irritated set of commands to get ready for school will result (7:10 A.M.). As the child begins to get dressed, he may do so in a disorganized fashion or slowly, resulting in more parental commands to get dressed appropriately (7:10–7:20 A.M.) (**avoidance of tasks that require sustaining mental effort, or potential skills deficit with planning/organization**). Because the child did not put his shoes in the front hall the night before, considerable time is spent looking for the shoes, which are eventually found in an unusual place for shoes, under the couch (**avoidance of a task that requires sustained mental effort: lack of organization skills related to putting shoes away**). The search for shoes includes a long lecture regarding the need to put things back where they belong because this happens all the time (7:20–7:25 A.M.). Once dressed, the child sits down for breakfast and because he is reaching to grab a magazine his sister is reading, he spills a full glass of orange juice all over the table and gets his parent's coat on the chair soaked and sticky (**attempting to gain tangible/gain attention**). His parent, now angry, yells at him to get his backpack and head outside toward the bus stop (7:30 A.M.). On the way to the bus stop at the corner, the parent scolds the child to "not bother the other kids like yesterday and just stand still!" The child, excited to see the other kids, gets upset when they do not reciprocate his excitement and teases one in front of the other parents, resulting in a reprimand from his parent and a number of cold stares from the other children's parents (**attempt to gain attention**). Finally, the bus arrives and the child's exasperated parent says, "Finally, the bus is here," and briskly walks back to the home without looking back (7:35 A.M.). . . . Then the child enters the classroom and instead of hanging up his coat and backpack in his cubby like the other children, he walks right back to the corner of the classroom where the class turtle is to look at it and see how it is doing (**avoidance of seatwork task**). As he is distracted by the turtle, the other classmates are sitting down and beginning their bellwork (7:50–8:00 A.M.). When the teacher notices him in the back of the room, the first thing she says to him is "Why aren't you ready? I hope today is not going to be another one of your days like yesterday because I am not in the mood to deal with it!" (8:00 A.M.).

Thus, as outlined above, there are multiple possible functions for the problematic behaviors, with the most common in this example being a desire to escape or avoid boring or tedious tasks, attempts to gain attention from adults and peers, and occasional attempts to gain something tangible for himself. One can also readily identify symptoms of DSM categories (e.g., ADHD, ODD), but it is also clear that these symptoms, in and of themselves, are less useful to a treatment provider than the functions of the behaviors. Ultimately, a practitioner has to try to figure out why the particular behavior "makes sense" from the point of view of the child. Once this is determined, it is much more likely that effective interventions can be developed and deployed.

In order to effectively support and intervene for this child, a strong treatment plan will necessarily incorporate components that address all these hypothesized functions. Furthermore, it is clear that the functions vary depending on the context—the function of the child's negative behaviors appears to be primarily escape/avoidance when confronted with tasks that are tedious or mundane; when the child is in social situations with peers, the function of the child's problematic behaviors appear to be more likely to have a functional goal of gaining attention. Treatment plans that do not include a means of addressing all functions of problematic behavior, or address the wrong function in a particular context (either because a single function is applied across all settings and situations or because it is hypothesized incorrectly), will fail to adequately address the referral problems. Therefore, as Chapter 3 outlines, a comprehensive functional behavioral assessment is one of the lynchpins of an effective approach for treating disruptive behavior disorders that occur in youth.

SUMMARY

This chapter outlines a way of thinking about disruptive behavior that may be somewhat antagonistic to current approaches and schools of thought that emphasize diagnosis using well-operationalized taxonomic systems. However, it is hoped that the rationale for deemphasizing diagnoses and emphasizing information and approaches that will foster effective treatment is one that resonates with practitioners whose job is not to name a disorder, but to treat it. In the chapter that follows, assessments that can be used to effectively integrate treatment and promote progress monitoring will be emphasized, consistent with the approach outlined herein.

CHAPTER 3

Overview of Assessment
for Informing Intervention

Within the functional assessment framework that will be emphasized throughout this book, evidence-based assessments for youth with ADHD, ODD, and CD are presented and reviewed. It is important when reviewing these measures that the reader remains mindful of the purposes of assessment, as the appropriate tool is likely to vary depending on the particular purpose of the assessment to be administered. Mash and Hunsley (2005) provide an excellent overview of the different purposes of assessment appropriate for youth including diagnosis and case formulation, screening, prediction, treatment planning, progress monitoring, and treatment outcome. These major assessment goals are reviewed for disruptive behavior disorders. Finally, some comments on the appropriate focus of assessments for disruptive behavior disorders, developmental considerations, and special considerations for assessment with particular groups are discussed.

PURPOSES OF ASSESSMENT

Prior to discussing the specific assessment approaches that are supported by evidence for the disruptive behavior disorders, it is useful to review the purposes of assessment. This is because the particular assessment tool must be appropriately aligned with the goal of the assessment conducted. Misalignment between the tool and the goal can result in confusing or inaccurate findings. This problem can be illustrated by a recent review of meta-analytic studies of ADHD psychosocial treatment outcome (Fabiano, Schatz, Aloe, Chacko, & Chronis-Tuscano, 2015). A meta-analysis is a review article that pulls together all the studies done on a particular topic and collapses the results together to illustrate the general effect across all the studies. Many meta-analyses of ADHD treatment outcomes have been conducted and the Fabiano and colleagues (2015) paper reviewed all the reviews. The review of meta-analyses of psychosocial ADHD treatments indicated effect sizes varied greatly. Within some meta-analytic reports psychosocial treatments had a negative, harmful effect on youth with ADHD (i.e., children in a control or no treatment group experienced better outcomes than those in the treatment group!) whereas in others there was a strong, therapeutic effect. One explanation for these discrepant results is that more positive results were obtained for meta-analyses that focused on appropriate target behaviors (e.g., social functioning, ADHD impairments) and that many of the negative effects were found for measures that were uncommonly targeted by ADHD interventions or unrelated to the core deficits for youth with ADHD (e.g., IQ, academic achievement test scores, internalizing symptoms).

A similar situation was encountered within the Multimodal Treatment Study for ADHD (MTA; MTA Cooperative Group, 1999) wherein youth with ADHD in psychosocial treatments did not significantly differ from a community comparison control group on measures of ADHD symptoms, but there were differences when one looked at functional outcomes such as parenting. These examples highlight the importance in aligning measures with the goal of the particular treatment conducted and the expected outcome of that treatment. For instance, in a treatment outcome study of daily report cards (DRCs) for youth with ADHD, significant and meaningful effects were found on measures of classroom behavior and academic productivity, but not for achievement in math or reading (Fabiano et al., 2010). Given the nature of the DRC intervention, which focuses mainly on modifying disruptive and academic enabling behavior, this result was expected; additional interventions to promote learning in academic content areas would likely be needed to obtain gains in this functional domain. However, it is easy to see how behavioral gains might be missed if an assessment battery included only achievement outcomes. Although this might seem to be an obvious example, compare it to current approaches in the country to use high-stakes achievement tests, administered on a single occasion within the school year, to determine the competency of teachers and student knowledge and one can perhaps begin an entirely new chapter on assessment approaches that have serious misalignment between the purpose of the measurement and the tool used to meet the assessment goal!

DISTINGUISHING BETWEEN FORMATIVE AND SUMMATIVE ASSESSMENTS

It is also important for individuals collecting assessments to be mindful of the two major roles of assessment: (1) formative assessment and (2) summative assessment. Formative assessment reflects the measurement of constructs that inform decisions about functional analyses, treatment planning, treatment modification, and ongoing versions of the educator's or parent's approach to working with the child. These assessments help inform the participants in the building, modifying, and evaluating of the treatment plan. Summative assessments, on the other hand, represent an overall evaluation. These summative assessments are more "black and white" in that they provide an overall, final accounting of progress. Daily quizzes children take to check for understanding might be conceptualized as formative assessments in a classroom whereas the final chapter test that is graded would represent a summative assessment.

By way of another example, in a kindergarten class, formative assessments might include a weekly measure of academic progress, such as how many letters and sounds can be identified by the child. Based on the results of this assessment, the teacher may modify instruction to target areas where the child still requires support. A summative assessment in this example would be the end-of-the-year academic reading test that determines whether it is appropriate to promote the child to the next grade. These two tests have quite different purposes, and it is clear the formative assessment has the teacher use the data collected from the measure to modify practice, whereas the summative assessment is somewhat removed from the student and teacher as it is solely evaluative. To shift to a behavioral example, office discipline referrals (ODRs) might be used as a formative assessment to determine how well a new schoolwide discipline plan is working. The location, grade level, and time of day of the referral could inform intervention efforts and program modifications. Summative assessments might include end-of-the-year reports to statewide authorities on the number of incidents that included violence or bullying. The purpose of these two behavioral measures is different, making one formative and one summative, even though the content of the measurement is similar. It is also easy to see how using a formative assessment for a summative purpose, or a summative assessment for a formative purpose, may cause difficulties in interpretation of outcomes or result in the reviewer of the information potentially making an inaccurate decision.

Given the emphasis in this book on functional outcomes, and an approach that includes continually gathering data to provide feedback on progress, inform modifications to treatment planning or measurement approaches, and indicate next directions, it should be the case that formative assessments occur much more often relative to summative assessment approaches. If a school or educator finds that summative assessments are occurring more frequently, or they are the only assessment being used, this is a potential cue to review the current measurement plan approach and ensure it appropriately aligns with the goals of the plan. It is also important to ensure that formative assessments are used in a manner consistent with their purpose: ODRs dutifully recorded and placed in a filing cabinet do not permit school administrators to effectively analyze these data to improve school functioning, for example, as they are not integrated together over time. Furthermore, although summative assessments are often emphasized in assessment planning, it is recommended that formative assessments should receive at least as much attention in schoolwide plans to assess behavior. In the sections that follow, formative and summative measures, for discrete purposes, are reviewed and evaluated. Recommendations for educators for integrating effective assessments for disruptive behaviors in schools are also provided.

EVIDENCE-BASED ASSESSMENTS FOR DISRUPTIVE BEHAVIOR DISORDERS

A number of assessment methods are available for identifying and diagnosing disruptive behavior disorders, including ADHD, ODD, and CD. The majority of these assessment methods ask a rater to provide information on the extent to which symptoms of these disorders are present, or whether specific behaviors are evident in the setting being rated.

Relatively fewer instruments are well established for assessing functional problems or for treatment planning, monitoring, and evaluation. This review is intended to provide practical advice on assessments for disruptive behavior disorders; the interested reader is referred to one of many comprehensive reviews that focuses on assessments for ADHD for more precise recommendations for specific measures (e.g., Barkley, 2015; Collett, Ohan, & Meyers, 2003a, 2003b; Johnston & Mah, 2008; Pelham et al., 2005).

ADHD assessments have predominantly focused on documenting behaviors consistent with ADHD symptoms (e.g., distractibility, impulsivity, difficulty sustaining attention), whereas general disruptive behavior disorder rating scales have been more likely to focus on specific problematic behaviors. The Eyberg Child Behavior Inventory (Robinson, Eyberg, & Ross, 1980), which is commonly used in samples of children with general disruptive behavior disorder problems, lists a number of problematic behaviors including throwing tantrums, noncompliance, and fighting, whereas ADHD rating scales often include the DSM symptoms of ADHD listed for the rater to endorse if present (e.g., Pelham, Gnagy, Greenslade, & Milich, 1992). In keeping with the practical approach to assessment and intervention advocated within this book, the disruptive behavior disorder rating scales will be emphasized, and specific, symptom-based rating scales are deemphasized. Perhaps a prescriber deciding whether or not medication should be used for ADHD would value an ADHD rating scale, but educators and parents who are charged with using positive behavioral supports for the child would still be left wanting for actionable data to use to plan intervention/treatment if a symptom-based rating scale was all that was used. This is because "fidgeting," "often is easily distractible by extraneous stimuli," and "plays or engages in leisure activities loudly" are not typical targets of treatment: they are neither face-valid nor socially valid. Reducing noncompliance, reducing teasing of peers and siblings, and the completion of assigned work are targets that are much more likely to be emphasized within treatment. Thus, in the review of specific assessments below, practical measures aligned with a functional emphasis in assessment will be spotlighted.

Screening

Leaders within the field of assessments for disruptive behavior disorders identify systematic screenings for disruptive behavior disorders to be among the most important achievements within the field in the last 50 years (Walker, 2015). Screening can accomplish many goals including the prevention of more serious disruptive or emotional problems that may develop if left unaddressed; permit lower-intensity, preventive interventions to be implemented effectively; and provide decision makers (e.g., teachers, principals, school psychologists) with actionable information from which to work. With respect to the last point, this is one of the key contributions of schoolwide positive behavioral supports. The School-Wide Information System (SWIS) is an assessment approach built into the PBIS frameworks used in schools. As such, it provides information on the extent to which teachers and others in the school are utilizing the program consistently, provides information on rule violations that occur (which ones, in what locations, at what time of day, by which grade level or classroom), and across settings and classrooms it provides a topography of problematic behavior within the setting. These data then inform intervention efforts. For example, if 75% of school rule violations or ODRs come from the second-grade team, professional development or support should be focused on those teachers and classes. If the majority of referrals outside the classroom are occurring within the cafeteria, then specific interventions to promote positive behaviors in that setting would be warranted (see, e.g., Fabiano et al., 2008). These targeted interventions would be difficult to appropriately employ without systematic screenings that inform practice.

Systematic screenings also address the ODR problem that can occur in schools. As noted above, outside of a systematic approach, ODRs can be very inconsistent in their use and evaluation. Some teachers would never refer a child to the office, save for the most serious behavioral infractions, due to a desire to keep discipline efforts within the classroom. At the other end of the continuum are teachers who refer children to the office for discipline for even minor behavioral concerns. In between these two types of teachers are those with different calibrations, just not at the extreme ends. Further complicating the interpretation of these ODRs, some teachers refer inconsistently across the school year or across behavioral concerns depending on the child or context. Thus, an administrator looking to use the ODR data to inform schoolwide behavioral interventions would be at a loss (and this is presuming these data are actually entered within a database that can be manipulated and scored; our experience is that these data are often detailed in a notebook at the secretary's desk or stored in an office filing cabinet on slips of paper).

Fortunately, systems like SWIS reduce some of the issues related to the limitations of ODR data. First, the data are collected within the context of an overall schoolwide plan related to discipline and positive behavioral supports. Second, the system is standardized within a computer program, and it provides the ability to score data quickly and accurately, producing output across an array of viewpoints (grade level, school setting, classroom, time of day, etc.). Third, the approach to collecting data is consistent across school years, permitting the ability to view patterns over the course of a single school year or across successive years. Because it is a standardized approach to collecting data, it also reduces inconsistencies that may arise when there is turnover in school leaders who are in charge of monitoring and managing the system.

Screening systems may alternatively include teacher or parent ratings of the school population. There are a number of approaches available that all require the rater to report on the students' behavior. Table 3.1 lists common assessments that can be used by teachers to screen for disruptive behavior in schools. Note, this is not an exhaustive list of screeners; it is only intended to provide an initial overview of the choices available for school practitioners. The measures listed in Table 3.1 have adequate indicators of reliability and validity, so school practitioners could reasonably choose any one for screening purposes depending on their own specific needs and preferences.

Although perhaps not as precise, screening can also be conducted using more nonobtrusive measures. These might include discipline referrals (see Form 3.1 at the end of this chapter for a sample referral sheet), a review of who is on the teacher's list of having incomplete homework assignments, or even a review of the messiness of the student's desk area and whether required materials (e.g., pencil, eraser) are present. An interesting study

TABLE 3.1. Examples of Screening Measures Appropriate for Use in School Settings to Identify Youth with or at Risk for Disruptive Behavior Disorders

Name	Age/grade targeted	Publisher's website	Number of items	Domains assessed	Scoring
Strengths and Difficulties Questionnaire (Goodman, 1997, 2001; Goodman & Goodman, 2009)	Ages 3–18	http://sdqinfo.org	25	Emotional symptoms; conduct problems, hyperactivity/inattention; peer relationship problems; prosocial behavior; total score	Measure yields five domains and a total score; no normative information available
Behavioral and Emotional Screening System (Kamphaus & Reynolds, 2007)	Ages 3–18	www.pearsonclinical.com	25	Single total score; validity indexes to identify overly negative or inconsistently rated responses	Norms available; T-scores and percentiles for the general U.S. population
Social, Academic, and Emotional Behavior Risk Screener (Kilgus, Chafouleas, & Riley-Tillman, 2013)	Grades K–12	http://ebi.missouri.edu/wp-content/uploads/2014/03/SAEBRS-Teacher-Rating-Scale-3.3.14.pdf (teacher version)	19	Social behavior; academic behavior; emotional behavior	No normative information available
Impairment Rating Scale (Evans et al., 2013; Fabiano et al., 2006)	Grades K–12	http://ccf.fiu.edu	6 items on teacher version; 7 items on parent version	Ratings across functional domains (relationship with peers, adults, academic progress, family/classroom functioning, self-esteem, sibling relationships) and overall impairment	Normative information available
Direct Behavior Rating (Chafouleas et al., 2013; Kilgus et al., 2014)	Grades K–8	http://directbehaviorratings.com	3	Ratings of disruptive behavior, academically engaged behavior, respectful behavior	No normative information available
Sutter–Eyberg Student Behavior Inventory—Revised (Eyberg & Pincus, 1999)	Ages 2–16	www4.parinc.com	38	Problem behavior frequency and intensity scores	Normative information available
Systematic Screening for Behavior Disorders (Walker, Severson, & Feil, 2014)	Grades 1–6	https://pacificnwpublish.com	33-item critical events checklist and 23-item frequency checklist for up to six students identified as at risk	Externalizing and internalizing behavior	Screening is conducted following teacher nomination of students of concern; no normative information available

by Atkins, Pelham, and Licht (1985) investigated which objective measures were best at identifying youth that teacher ratings indicated had ADHD. Teacher-identified youth with or without ADHD were correctly classified 83% of the time using a combination of six objective measures that included the percent of seatwork correctly completed, whether the child exhibited interruptive behavior (talking to self, verbal intrusion), whether the child sat at his or her desk during the observation, and whether the child was prepared for class (has a pencil and eraser at the desk). This study suggests that brief direct behavior ratings (Chafouleas et al., 2013) related to these behaviors may be viable screeners for identifying youth with disruptive behavior disorders, and that they may identify youth effectively relative to more intensive and costly measures.

An advantage of this direct behavior rating approach using a smaller number of items should be strongly considered in screening efforts. Consider a 30-item rating scale completed by a teacher for 25 children in the class. This is a total of 750 items that must be rated and then scored and interpreted. A five-item rating scale completed for the same class would represent only 125 total checkmarks the teacher would need to complete (not to mention the cognitive effort that needs to go into reading each item, thinking about the specific child and the specific behavior, and then making a decision regarding what evaluation to provide), which represents an 84% reduction in the amount of ratings that need to be completed. This more efficient approach is likely to be better received by educators, and it may also result in more meaningful ratings as it should reduce rater fatigue. An alternative approach that also increases the efficiency of screening ratings has been advocated by Walker and colleagues (2014) wherein the teacher first nominates the top three children with disruptive behavior disorder concerns, and then the more extensive screener is completed for this smaller, focused grouping of children. Either approach is likely to be more efficient, so educators and school psychologists are encouraged to think about using screening methods that are consistent with the expressed purpose of behavioral screenings: to reliably identify the youth most in need of further functional assessments so as to inform treatment that will reduce impairment from disruptive behavior. Simply filling out lengthy ratings for all children in the school to obtain data on the extent to which disruptive behavior is present is not part of this expressed goal for screening.

Diagnosis

Given the emphasis in this book on functional assessments rather than diagnostic approaches, this section is purposely brief. Educators can readily "diagnose" children who have reading problems, behavior problems, or social problems (e.g., Gresham, Reschly, & Carey, 1987). Therefore, it is a bit confusing why diagnosis has been increasingly emphasized as something important for youth with disruptive behavior disorders in school settings. It is notable that there are no special education categories for "ADHD," making it unclear what goal is achieved by educators emphasizing ADHD diagnostic procedures. Perhaps an insidious reason for this diagnostic emphasis is that if a child has a diagnosis of ADHD, he or she is more likely to have medication prescribed. A consequence of this emphasis on diagnosis is a reduction in assessment time dedicated to the other purposes of assessment, described below, that focus on intervention planning and outcomes. Thus, it is the position of this book that diagnosis should be completed as quickly and efficiently as possible, while maintaining accuracy, if it is a necessary purpose for assessment, so as to leave more time for functional analysis, treatment planning, and progress monitoring.

It may seem intuitive to complete diagnosis quickly and then spend time on treatment, but this is not always the case in the field. We recently began working with teenagers with ADHD who were learning to drive. One of our challenges was a need to establish a clear diagnosis of "ADHD, combined type" according to DSM criteria, for research purposes (in research environments diagnoses are important so that the sample can be characterized precisely enough to permit replication of the experiment using a similar participant group). In order to help document the age-of-onset criterion for ADHD (at that time ADHD symptoms had to be present and impairing before the age of 7), we asked families to bring in any old reports, individualized education plans, and other documentation related to the ADHD diagnosis. It was not uncommon for families to bring in large accordion files or binders full of assessment results, with some reports going back to early childhood. The research staff dutifully photocopied all these reports so the study doctors could review them in their diagnostic review for each case. One thing that struck the doctors during the review was that there was often very clear consensus across the reports starting from early in childhood and progressing through adolescence that the child had clear and impairing disruptive behaviors. Something that was disappointing about the information was what was lacking: follow-up reports that included treatment plans, summaries, and outcomes. Many of the children had received multiple diagnostic reports but had had limited documentation in the realm of treatment; presumably this was because the provider completed the diagnostic assessment but then ended clinical contact or referred out to a pediatrician or school for follow-up intervention. This was disappointing because it was likely that the reason parents were obtaining the diagnostic report in the first place was to use it to get help. As professionals in the field, this example serves as a warning that diagnosis should not be viewed as a summative assessment, but rather as a first step in an ongoing series of formative assessments to provide information that can be used in a progressive fashion in support of intervention.

With that in mind, papers on evidence-based assessment for disruptive behavior disorders suggest that the diagnostic approach can be straightforward and sufficient information can be readily obtained to inform diagnostic decision making. Pelham and colleagues (2005) reported that results from brief rating scales completed by parents and teachers on the presence and severity of ADHD symptoms were comparable to more lengthy structured interviews. McMahon and Frick (2005) also list rating scales as an evidence-based approach to identifying youth with conduct problems, as most broad-band rating scales include a youth self-, parent-, and teacher-report version. Thus, once the child is identified as having clinically significant levels of symptoms, professionals should not "beat a dead horse" by administering other measures to identify clinically significant levels of symptoms. Rather, as both McMahon and Frick and Pelham and colleagues emphasize, assessments past that point should focus on obtaining information on the nature, function, frequency, and intensity of the behavior; the settings where it is present; and the resultant impairment from the behaviors. These data are typically formative, they are part of an assessment of function, and they directly support treatment planning efforts.

Functional Assessment and Intervention Planning

Professionals should have the goal in mind that all assessments will focus on informing intervention. For instance, we have often used the Impairment Rating Scale (Fabiano et al., 2006; available for download at *http://ccf.fiu.edu/for-families/resources-for-parents/ printable-information/impairment_rating_scales.pdf*) in our clinical work. It provides a quantitative rating on a continuum of need for services that reliably classifies youth with disruptive behavior versus those who are not identified as having these problems. For treatment planning, it also asks parents and teachers to provide a narrative description of the child's functioning and any impairment in major life domains (i.e., peer relationships, group functioning in the family or classroom, relationship with adults such as parents or the teacher, academic progress, self-esteem, and overall). These narratives often are good starting points for identifying specific targets for treatment goals and objectives. For example, a parent might write, "I am concerned my child does not seem to keep friends. I notice when he plays with others in the home he is quite bossy. He frequently comes home from school complaining of teasing and bullying. I notice he has a hard time reading social cues such as when another child is getting frustrated with his overbearing approach." A teacher might write under the academic progress topic, "The teen often comes to class without his required books and notebook, and usually not even a pen. I think he is a capable student, but I have yet to receive a completed homework assignment, which is a large drag on his grade. I also find myself correcting him to get back on task when students are supposed to work individually." Based on these notes, clinically rich details on functioning become clearer, and they assist the treatment planner in addressing the very areas that parents and teachers identify as in need of help and support. This facilitates the first step in functional behavioral analysis: the identification of *target behaviors*. Target behaviors represent the areas of functioning that need to be addressed within treatment in order to make meaningful improvements for the youth. These target behaviors may be reduced or increased through treatment. For instance, interruptions during class lectures would be a target behavior that interventions would reduce, and organization of a school locker would be a target behavior that would be increased.

Once identified, the target behaviors have to be carefully operationalized to ensure that the identification and evaluation of the presence and absence of the behavior is done consistently across raters/observers as well as across time. Thus, behaviors such as "on-task" or "disruptive" are poor target behaviors unless they are backed by carefully constructed operational definitions that provide information on what does and does not represent the behavior. Targeted behaviors to improve such as "organization" will often need to be broken down into component parts to ensure that the behaviors that represent "organization" are appropriately identified, tracked, and evaluated (e.g., Evans et al., 2009). Operational definitions of targeted behaviors may sometimes include specific examples to orient the raters, they may include contrasting examples, or they may be illustrated via videotaped vignettes

(Pelham, Greiner, & Gnagy, 2008; Schlientz et al., 2009). Form 3.2 at the end of this chapter enables the practitioner to label the target behavior and operationalize it in concrete, observable, behavioral terms.

Functional behavioral analysis is the next part of intervention planning (Crone, Hawken, & Horner, 2015; Crone & Horner, 2003; Steege & Watson, 2009). Following the identification and operationalization of targeted behaviors, an analysis of the situations and settings where the behavior occurs, development of ideas about hypothesized functions for the targeted behaviors, and a decision regarding the function of the behavior should be carried out. Essentially, the practitioner must attempt to figure out why a behavior is occurring—what motivation might be behind it, why does it occur, and what might be serving to maintain it. Typically, a problem behavior will seem to make no sense to others, but in order for a behavior to be exhibited repeatedly by a youth, there must be some reason for it to make sense from the youth's point of view. After the first step in identifying the target behaviors, the next steps include interviewing the teacher and other adults involved with the child to identify situations where the behavior occurs and does not occur, identify the situations and contexts that either improve or exacerbate the problematic behavior, and identify the antecedents (i.e., triggers, precipitating events) and consequences (positive and negative outcomes) of the behavior. These contextual and potentially maintaining variables can help the practitioner begin to develop a hypothesis of the reason (e.g., escape/avoidance; gain to self via tangible rewards or attention; self-stimulation; skills deficit) the target behavior is being exhibited by the child.

Using Form 3.3, a school psychologist or other professional could identify a target behavior and conduct a functional behavioral assessment. In this approach the team first identifies a targeted behavior, or a set of behaviors, that is then analyzed to determine possible function. Figure 3.1 illustrates how this form might be completed for a child with insubordination in the classroom. The professional would interview a teacher or team of teachers, conduct observations of the behaviors, identify the antecedents and consequences of the behavior, describe variables that might maintain or increase/decrease the intensity of the behavior, and define a hypothesized function for the behavior.

As is clear from the description of a functional behavioral assessment, this is not a small or rapid task. It is one that takes considerable effort and the collective brain power of a number of individuals who are working to support the child. Importantly, however, these assessment activities directly lead to intervention. For the teen described in Figure 3.1 the determination was made that the insubordinate behavior was exhibited to avoid tasks that were disliked. In this case, intervention approaches were developed to prevent the teen from avoiding tasks that were disliked through insubordination. In partnership with the parent, all academic activities that were not completed during the class day were instead completed after school during a time the teen typically spent with friends playing videogames. This change in the management of the activities resulting in the teen having the choice to avoid academics during the school day, but also coupled that decision with the consequence of missing time together with friends. Additional information collected suggested that the teen highly valued peer attention, and he did not want to stand out negatively in front of peers. Therefore, the initial intervention approach to ensure the teen was

1. Target behavior (Define the behavior in concrete, observable terms. Be sure to define only a single behavior; repeat the process for other, distinct behaviors.): Insubordination: The child refuses to comply with a direct command or request within 5 seconds of it being issued.

2. List all the situations where the behavior occurs: Demands placed on him. Demands from the social studies teacher and from unfamiliar adults (e.g., cafeteria staff) are especially likely to be met with insubordination.

   List all the situations where the behavior does not occur: During specials classes, football practice

3. Describe other situations, people, or contexts that make the behavior worse or better: When friends are around, insubordination toward adults is worse. Demands that include handwriting also are likely to be followed by the behavior.

4. What happens before the behavior occurs (i.e., antecedents or triggers)? Demand to begin writing; teen feels the behavioral request is too demanding.

5. What happens after the behavior occurs (i.e., consequences, rewards, punishments, something else)? Teen avoids demand; teen is sent to the disciplinarian's office and leaves class; teen receives positive attention from peers (e.g., giggling); adult reprimand and increasing demands.

6. Describe any attempts to modify or control identified antecedents and consequences. Results? Teachers used "natural consequences" for a week where the teen could choose to complete work, or not, and teachers did not put demands on him. No work was done that week.

7. Hypothesized function:
   ☐ Attention from adults   ☐ Attention from peers   ☐ Gain to self—tangible   ☐ Gain to self—privilege
   ☑ Escape/avoid   ☐ Self-stimulation   ☐ Other (describe): _____

8. Ideas for intervention based on the hypothesized function in (7) above: The teen is exhibiting the behavior to escape demands, especially those that include writing. He does accept demands in other situations (e.g., football practice). We will work with the coach to defer all refused tasks until after school, and he will not be allowed to join practice until he has finished all work expected for the day. When all work is completed, then he can join practice.

FIGURE 3.1. Example of a completed Functional Behavioral Assessment and Intervention Planning Form.

unable to avoid work through disruptive, insubordinate behavior was developed based on the functional assessment conducted.

Measurement of Integrity and Fidelity

Even the best intervention in the world won't be any good if it is not implemented as intended. An example of this occurred when I was in a classroom the other day. The school had invested in an expensive "smart board" that had a projector, was linked to student clickers that could permit real-time formative assessments, and had a number of other "bells and whistles" that were supposed to promote student learning. The teachers all went to a training to learn how to use the new technology. When I was in the classroom conducting an observation, the teacher, who was exasperated because she could not get the technology to work, had taped a large piece of poster paper to the smartboard and was using it as a simple (yet expensive!) easel. This is a good example of how the best-laid plans can go awry, with the initial intentions of an intervention plan drifting or changing due to circumstance or technical difficulties. Therefore, procedures for ensuring plans have integrity and fidelity are critical in the treatment of disruptive behaviors in schools. This is especially critical in the realm of interventions for youth with disruptive behaviors, where school psychologists or other professionals may consult with teachers or other school staff as indirect/consultative intervention providers, with the expectations that teachers or school staff then directly implement the intervention. Although consultants may craft elegant intervention plans, they should be mindful that the follow-through of these plans is often modest, with many educators not implementing the plan at all following a consultation meeting (Martens & Ardoin, 2002)!

Fabiano, Chafouleas, and colleagues (2014) define integrity as whether the implementation of the assessments and interventions occurred as intended. A related construct, fidelity, refers to the quality with which the intervention was delivered to the targeted child or classroom. An example provided in Fabiano and colleagues suggest that the use of a radio can be used as an analogy for the assessment of integrity and fidelity. Tuning the radio to the correct station is like an intervention implemented with integrity. The fidelity of the intervention is represented by the song being clearly transmitted and free of static without a disc jockey talking over it. As interventions are developed and implemented, school professionals should create checklists to operationalize the active ingredients of the intervention, the person(s) responsible for implementing each aspect of the intervention, how the quality of the intervention will be addressed and rated, and whether there are any components that are proscribed (i.e., would not be a part of the active intervention). Form 3.2 provides a brief example of a checklist that can be utilized to ensure a DRC is appropriately created with consultant support to a teacher.

Intervention Outcome

An additional important target of assessment relates to the measurement of the intervention outcome. This is an approach interwoven into the fabric of schools. Report cards are one obvious example of an assessment of academic intervention outcome. Statewide assessments could also be conceptualized as summative assessments to evaluate the learning that has happened due to academic instruction. Teachers who track the number of books read and provide a pizza party once a certain target is reached are also assessing outcome (and progress monitoring if they are tracking steps toward the target along the way). When one considers behavior disorders, outcome assessments are also frequently utilized. Many of the screening measures in Table 3.1 can also be used as measures of outcome. These measures, if used for screening, can also serve as pretreatment indicators of functioning. Readministering the measure would help the educators and other involved professionals know whether the interventions that were implemented improved behavior.

A key issue in intervention outcome relates to the social validity of the outcome. Changing by a fraction of a point on a symptom rating scale or reducing a score on a screening instrument might be important, but only inasmuch as it represents functional improvement. If a child receives better scores on a measure, but does not improve in the key areas of functioning (i.e., relationships with peers and adults, academic progress, group functioning), then these changes and improvements become less compelling. Importantly, these key areas of functioning are the places where improvement is needed if the child is going to experience positive outcomes in the future. They are also the areas that educators and parents care the most about, so they should be primary targets of outcome assessments. Significantly, the magnitude of treatment effects varies across areas of functioning. For instance, a recent review illustrated that children with ADHD across studies were likely to improve in social behaviors following a psychosocial treatment, but improvement in ADHD symptoms was less consistent across studies (Fabiano et al., 2015). On the one hand, one might view this outcome as negative because improvement was not observed across domains. However, on the other hand, the picture could be viewed as much brighter because improvement in social behavior is much more important than obtaining a reduced overall score on a symptom rating scale. This example underscores the importance of thoughtful outcome assessment planning.

SUMMARY

This chapter outlines some effective approaches for assessing disruptive behavior, taking into consideration that there are multiple goals of assessment. Practitioners interested in the effective assessment of disruptive behavior must ensure that there is alignment between the goals of the assessment and the tools used to meet these goals. Furthermore, it is recommended that the field return to an emphasis on formative assessments that are much more aligned with treatment tasks and efforts, and reserve summative assessments for research outcome studies and less frequent checks of progress. Finally, across screening, treatment planning, measures of integrity and fidelity, and treatment outcome, practitioners should be mindful that the purpose of assessments is ultimately to inform intervention that will build competencies and reduce the impaired functioning of youth with disruptive behaviors.

Office Discipline Referral (ODR) Sheet

Student Name: _____ Date: _____

Teacher Name: _____ Time: _____

Reason for Referral:

☐ Aggression with intent to do significant harm (i.e., would typically result in mark or bruise)

☐ Engaging in dangerous situation

☐ Insubordination

☐ Possession of a dangerous item

☐ Property damage

☐ Stealing

☐ Sexual harassment

☐ Swearing/obscene language

☐ Other (please indicate): _____

Comments: _____

_____

_____

_____

_____

_____

Location: _____

_____

_____

Office Response:

☐ Time-out   ☐ Student conference

☐ Phone call home   ☐ Letter home

☐ Sent home for the day   ☐ Parent conference

☐ Suspension   ☐ Other: _____

Comments: _____

_____

_____

_____

_____

_____

Treatment Integrity and Fidelity Checklist for Establishing a Daily Report Card (DRC)

This form can be completed by a supervisor or as a self-report checklist.

Objectives:

☐ To begin to build a cooperative and collaborative relationship with the teacher.

☐ To introduce the DRC.

☐ To identify target behaviors that can be operationally defined and included on the DRC.

Procedures:

☐ Review the process for establishing a DRC with teacher.

☐ Work with the teacher to create appropriate targets for the child.

☐ Complete the template for a preliminary DRC and review the formatting and procedures for the plan (e.g., will target behaviors be evaluated after each class or in the A.M./P.M.?).

☐ Explain to teacher that he or she should describe DRC targets to the child as well as the home rewards component.

☐ Schedule a follow-up with the teacher for 1 week following the initiation of the plan.

Postvisit Procedures:

☐ Complete a contact note for the meeting.

☐ Call parents to inform them when the DRC will be starting.

Rating of Alliance with Teacher:

1	2	3	4	5	6	7
Poor			Neutral			Excellent

Communication:

1	2	3	4	5	6	7
Discouraging, focused on negative			Neutral			Encouraging, focused on positive

Functional Behavioral Assessment and Intervention Planning Form

Use the form below to conduct a functional behavioral assessment of target behaviors. Use a separate form for each behavior.

1. Target behavior (Define the behavior in concrete, observable terms. Be sure to define only a single behavior; repeat the process for other, distinct behaviors.): _____

   _____

2. List all the situations where the behavior occurs: _____

   _____

   List all the situations where the behavior does not occur: _____

   _____

3. Describe other situations, people, or contexts that make the behavior worse or better: _____

   _____

   _____

4. What happens before the behavior occurs (i.e., antecedents or triggers)? _____

   _____

   _____

5. What happens after the behavior occurs (i.e., consequences, rewards, punishments, something else)? _____

   _____

   _____

6. Describe any attempts to modify or control identified antecedents and consequences. Results? ____

   _____

   _____

7. Hypothesized function:

   ☐ Attention from adults ☐ Attention from peers ☐ Gain to self—tangible ☐ Gain to self—privilege

   ☐ Escape/avoid   ☐ Self-stimulation   ☐ Other (describe): _____

8. Ideas for intervention based on the hypothesized function in (7) above: _____

   _____

   _____

   _____

   _____

   _____

   _____

CHAPTER 4

Parent Training Interventions

The cornerstone of most effective interventions for a child with a disruptive behavior disorder will be a parent training program. Parent training programs typically teach effective strategies for promoting appropriate child behavior using well-manualized approaches and emphasize the fundamentals of behavior change through rewards, punishments, and modeling, as well as basic information about disruptive behavior disorders. Parents are given assigned readings and are taught standard behavioral techniques such as those shown in Table 4.1 (Barkley, 2013; Cunningham, Bremner, & Secord, 1998; Eyberg & Funderburk, 2011; Forehand & Long, 1996; Patterson, 1975a; Webster-Stratton, 1997, 2005). Typical clinical parent training programs include a series of eight to 16 weekly sessions for the initial training, and the intervention is continued as long as is necessary, with programs for maintenance and relapse prevention typically built in. Parent training is accomplished individually or in groups, with weekly assignments given to parents to track behavior and practice techniques with their children between sessions. The behavioral parent training (BPT) topics listed in Table 4.1 can best be thought of as a good start, as there are additional topics that may be covered either in a group or individually. Coverage for many of these topics (e.g., time-out) may span multiple sessions.

General reviews on BPT support its use for children described as ADHD, antisocial, or disruptive (e.g., Brestan & Eyberg, 1998; Evans et al., 2013; Eyberg et al., 2008; Lundahl, Risser, & Lovejoy, 2006; Pelham & Fabiano, 2008; Serketich & Dumas, 1996). Meta-analyses also yield positive effects for BPT. Corcoran and Dattalo (2006) reported effect sizes of 0.40 and 0.36 for ADHD and externalizing symptoms, respectively, in their meta-analysis of between-group studies of parent-involved treatments for ADHD. Lundahl and colleagues (2006) reviewed between-group BPT studies for children described as disruptive and reported effect sizes ranging from 0.42 to 0.53 for child and parent outcomes following intervention. Serketich and Dumas (1996) included only group design studies and reported an overall effect size of 0.86 for BPT interventions. Fabiano and colleagues (2009)

TABLE 4.1. Typical Content of Sessions for a Parent Training Program for Attention-Deficit/Hyperactivity Disorder

1. Overview of behavior management principles and how disruptive behaviors can be maintained through functional relationships.
2. Establishing a home–school DRC/rewarding the DRC.
3. Attending, rewarding appropriate behavior, and planned ignoring of minor, inappropriate behaviors (e.g., whining).
4. Giving effective commands and instructions.
5. Time-out/privilege removal procedures.
6. Establishing and enforcing rules.
7. When . . . then contingencies.
8. Home point system—reward and response cost.
9. Enforcing contingencies outside of the home/planning ahead.
10. Arranging structured play dates.
11. Maintenance of program after weekly therapist contact ends.

completed a meta-analysis across the ADHD treatment literature and reported a weighted effect size within the large range for between-group studies, with substantial effect sizes from studies that measured parenting using objective observations of specific parenting behaviors (effect size = 2.51). Thus, this treatment approach results in moderate to substantial improvement for children with a variety of disruptive behavior problems.

BPT PROGRAMS FOR CHILDREN WITH DISRUPTIVE BEHAVIOR DISORDERS

There are currently a number of well-validated, manualized parent training programs available for clinicians to implement. These programs are typically based on the work of Patterson and Gullion (1968), Hanf (1969), and K. D. and S. G. O'Leary and their lab at Stony Brook University (e.g., O'Leary & Pelham, 1978; O'Leary, Pelham, Rosenbaum, & Price, 1976). Below, a nonexhaustive sample of parenting programs used for children with disruptive behavior disorders is reviewed, including a program description and current evidence for the program effectiveness in order to provide exemplars of best practice.

Defiant Children

The Defiant Children program (Barkley, 2013) is manualized, and includes 10 steps for addressing the behavior problems associated with children with ADHD. Topics covered include psychoeducational information on behavior, using attending strategies to promote appropriate behavior, token economies, time-out, planning ahead for behavior in public places, and using a school–home DRC. Each session has a well-described set of issues and topics for the clinician to present, discuss, and obtain feedback about from the parent(s). Furthermore, there is a reproducible handout that summarizes each session and lists the tasks for the parent to attempt during the week. The program can be administered to individual families or to groups.

Defiant Children has been evaluated in multiple studies. Anastopoulos, Shelton, DuPaul, and Guevremont (1993) administered the Defiant Children parenting intervention individually to families in a treatment group ($n = 19$) and compared outcomes to a wait-list group ($n = 15$). Treated families demonstrated improvements in ratings of child ADHD symptoms and parent-reported feelings of competence and stress, and these effects were maintained at a 2-month follow-up appointment. Barkley and colleagues (2000) also evaluated the Defiant Children program, both alone and in combination with a school-based intervention, relative to a no treatment condition with kindergarten children at risk for ADHD and other disruptive behaviors. In this study, the parent training program produced no significant effects, though 35% of parents in the parent training only group attended zero sessions. When the parenting training alone group and parenting training plus school intervention groups were collapsed together, only 13% of parents attended 60% or more of the sessions. Thus, although the program did not result in statistically significant improvements, it is possible that any potential effects were diluted by the finding that the majority of families did not receive the parent training treatment dose as intended. These findings highlight the importance of engagement efforts to promote attendance within BPT programs, as discussed further in Chapter 9.

There is also an extension of the Defiant Children program for adolescents called Defiant Teens. The content of the program targeting adolescents is similar to the child-focused program, but includes important modifications for a teenager with ADHD. These include teaching behavior management strategies to parents that are appropriate for adolescents. Following the behavior management strategy sessions (Sessions 1–9), which include only the parents, the adolescent then joins the intervention and a series of sessions to introduce and teach problem-solving communication training (Sessions 10–18; Robin & Foster, 1989).

This program has been evaluated in two studies conducted by Barkley and colleagues (Barkley, Edwards, Laneri, Fletcher, & Metevia, 2001; Barkley, Guevremont, Anastopoulos, & Fletcher, 1992). In the initial study (Barkley et al., 1992), the Defiant Teens program behavior management strategies were compared to problem-solving communication training and structural family therapy groups. Results indicated improved functioning in child domains, parent domains, and parent–child interactions, and groups did not significantly differ. Barkley and colleagues (2001) compared the Defiant Teens program (nine sessions of behavior management strategies followed by nine sessions of problem-solving communication strategies) to 18 sessions of problem-solving communication training alone. Both groups evinced improvements in teen and parent functioning, and did not differ. However, significantly more families persisted (i.e., did not drop out of the intervention) with the Defiant Teens treatment relative to problem-solving communication training alone.

Fabiano and colleagues (2011) recently adapted the Defiant Teens program to focus on driving outcomes for youth with ADHD and related disruptive behavior disorders. Teenage drivers are among the riskiest on the road, and, compared to typically developing teens, teens with ADHD are at significantly greater risk for most negative driving outcomes (i.e., citations, accidents, injuries, death; Fabiano & Schatz, 2014). In this study, parents attended an initial 45-minute session to learn and decide how to apply the BPT content within the Defiant Teens curriculum. In parallel, the teens were learning problem-solving and communication skills. Following the initial 45-minute session, parents and teens joined together to complete a problem-solving task that included the creation of a contingency contract to support safe driving behaviors. Initial pilot work suggested that this was a feasible and promising approach for working with novice drivers who had disruptive behavior disorders. Notably, compliance with treatment sessions was uniformly high for parents and teens, perhaps because each treatment constituent was motivated to engage with the intervention: parents were anxious to provide additional supports for the teen with whom they were concerned, and teens were eager to engage because they saw the intervention as a mechanism to potentially increase driving privileges. This suggests that the initiation to driving may be a good entry point for practitioners interested in employing parent–teen interventions during the high school years.

Community Parent Education Program

The Community Parent Education Program (COPE; Cunningham, Bremner, & Secord, 1998) is implemented with large groups of parents (approximately 20–30) using a coping–modeling–problem-solving approach. COPE includes 16 sessions as well as procedures for booster sessions and a concurrently run child social skills group. In contrast to a didactic approach to parent training, the leader does not provide prescriptive information; rather, the leader promotes group members' generation of their own solutions. In this approach, parents view videotapes of exaggerated parenting errors, discuss these mistakes and their potential impact with other parents, and formulate solutions for the situation. The leader serves as a facilitator for this process, and models the group members' proposed solutions in addition to encouraging the group members' rehearsal of the behavioral strategies in role-play exercises.

Available evidence supports the efficacy of COPE. Cunningham, Bremner, and Boyle (1995) compared COPE to an individual-focused, clinic-based parenting program and a wait list. In this study, COPE participants reported more reductions in home-based child behavior problems relative to the other two groups, and these gains were maintained through the 6-month follow-up. Furthermore, COPE participants demonstrated improved problem-solving skills, measured by the number of solutions offered during discussions. Families facing barriers to parent-training participation (e.g., those with more serious child management problems) were also more likely to participate in COPE relative to those in the individual, clinic-based program. The COPE style of parent training was also adapted for adolescents with ADHD, and a preliminary study suggests positive outcomes when the program targets this older age group (McCleary & Ridley, 1999).

The COPE style of parent training has been shown to be superior to a traditional didactic approach on measures of engagement such as attendance and arrival on time for sessions, homework completion, and interaction with other parents in-session (Cunningham et al., 1993). COPE lends itself well to engaging large groups, potentially disenfranchised groups within BPT efforts (i.e., fathers; see Chapter 9), and it is relatively easy to train group leaders in this effective approach to intervention. The group parent training approach is also highly economical because a single facilitator can treat upward of 20 families simultaneously within this format. Another advantage of the COPE model is that when families work together within subgroups, every member of the group has an opportunity to talk and provide substantive responses, something that may not always happen in a large group where a few members dominate the conversation. Thus, the COPE model for parent training is more efficient and potentially more effective across families.

Parent–Child Interaction Therapy

Parent–Child Interaction Therapy (PCIT; Eyberg & Boggs, 1998; Eyberg & Robinson, 1982) is typically administered individually to a family and follows two stages. In the first stage, child-directed interaction (CDI), the therapist works with the parent to develop and foster a positive parent–child relationship through positive social attention, use of labeled praise, and ignoring of minor negative behaviors. In the second stage, parent-directed interaction (PDI), parents work to increase appropriate behavior and decrease negative behavior in their child through antecedent control (e.g., use of clear instructions/commands) and consequences (e.g., time-out). Parents begin the CDI portion of treatment in a meeting with the therapist to introduce the topic and then subsequent sessions include parent–child interactions that are observed by the therapist and feedback/coaching is provided based on these observations, often online using a bug-in-the-ear device. Parents continue to participate in the observed interactions until mastery of the skill is demonstrated. Once a skill is mastered, another CDI skill is introduced, and PDI sessions follow after the CDI sessions are successfully completed.

Most of the published research on PCIT implemented the treatment with young children (i.e., 3–5 years old) with disruptive behavior disorders (i.e., ADHD, ODD, and CD). Because of the high rates of comorbidity among the disruptive behavior disorders, many of the children in these studies were diagnosed with multiple disruptive behavior disorder problems, suggesting this approach is effective even for youth with multiple disruptive behaviors that require treatment. Schuhmann, Foote, Eyberg, Boggs, and Algina (1998) investigated the effectiveness of PCIT with families with a child with ODD, and 66% of the sample also met diagnostic criteria for ADHD. Families were randomly assigned to PCIT or a wait-list control condition. Families in the PCIT group demonstrated improvement on the proximal outcome of parenting skills as well as improvements in the distal outcome of child behavior. In another study on the efficacy of PCIT, in which approximately 75% of participants had ADHD, Eisenstadt, Eyberg, McNeil, Newcomb, and Funderburk (1993) reported improvements in child behavior, parenting, and parenting stress. Follow-up evaluations of PCIT suggest treatment effects persist up to 6 years after the intervention (Hood & Eyberg, 2003).

Triple-P Positive Parenting Program

The Triple-P Positive Parenting Program (Sanders, 1999) is a tiered program that includes preventive and targeted interventions for parents. There are five levels of the Triple-P program: the Universal Triple P (targeting all parents), Selective Triple P (helping parents with a specific behavioral concern, e.g., toilet training), Primary Care Triple P (one to four sessions that deal with a specific behavioral concern), Standard Triple P (a course of parenting sessions for parents of children with severe behavior problems), and Enhanced Triple P (an intensive course of parenting sessions that targets child behavior as well as family-related problems). The Triple-P program is well validated and has been disseminated across the world. Many children with a chronic disruptive behavior disorder are likely to require the more intensive level of treatment in the Triple-P program, such as the Standard or Enhanced program.

The Triple-P program has been evaluated in samples of children with disruptive behavior disorders. Hoath and Sanders (2002) randomly assigned families to the Enhanced Triple-P program or a wait-list group. Following treatment, parents in the treatment group reported improved child-related outcomes and use of parenting strategies. Importantly, intervention effects were maintained when assessed at a 3-month follow-up evaluation. In another study using a sample of preschoolers with ADHD-related behaviors, Bor, Sanders, and Markie-Dadds (2002) compared an enhanced parent training condition to a standard condition, and both groups were compared to a wait-list control group. Results indicated both BPT programs resulted in improved child behavior and increased parenting skills and sense of competence. These gains were maintained at 1-year follow-up, and there were no significant differences between the two parent training interventions. Both studies support the effectiveness of the Triple-P parenting program with families with a child with ADHD.

The Incredible Years

The Incredible Years program (Webster-Stratton, 1997, 2005) includes a Basic parenting program appropriate for children ages 2–10 that focuses on parenting skills, an Advanced parenting program that includes training in interpersonal skills (e.g., anger management, communication), and an Education parenting program to assist with promoting the child's academic success. During the programs, parents view videotapes of parents in typical parenting situations, and then discuss the videotapes, including what they liked about the parent's approach and what they might have done differently. The Basic program is offered to groups of parents in 2-hour weekly sessions and lasts approximately 14 weeks. Fourteen additional sessions of the Advanced curriculum, or six additional sessions of the Education curriculum, may be offered following completion of the Basic program.

The Incredible Years has been evaluated in a number of empirical studies (see Webster-Stratton, 2005, for a review). Similar to the literature on PCIT, most children included in the studies were diagnosed with ODD or CD, but given comorbidity rates it is likely that many children also met criteria for ADHD. Webster-Stratton, Reid, and Hammond (2004) reported results from a study that randomly assigned families to receive parent training alone, child social skills training alone, parent or child training plus teacher training, or parent, child, and teacher training. Results demonstrated that any condition that included parent training resulted in improved parenting skills (e.g., use of fewer negative/coercive parenting strategies) and fewer child behavior problems at posttreatment. Children in this study were followed up 2 years later (Reid, Webster-Stratton, & Hammond, 2003), and approximately three-quarters of them were reported to be functioning within the normal range on a standard assessment.

When response to The Incredible Years is investigated, results suggest that children with ADHD and comorbid ODD or CD respond well to the intervention. Hartman, Stage, and Webster-Stratton (2003) found that children with ADHD and a comorbid externalizing disorder improved in response to parent training *more than* conduct-problem children without comorbid ADHD. Webster-Stratton has also demonstrated through multiple controlled trials that The Incredible Years curriculum is an effective approach for improving parenting skills and strategies, child behavior, and family functioning.

Parent Management Training—The Oregon Model

Parent Management Training—The Oregon Model (PMTO; Forgatch & Patterson, 2005; Patterson & Forgatch, 2005) represents a well-developed and empirically validated parent training approach that helps parents utilize effective parenting strategies. It directly addresses and reduces a coercive process within the family (see Chapter 2); targets problems within and across the family, school, and peer settings; and directly aims to build functional competencies. PMTO is appropriate for parents of children between the ages of 2 and 18 and it can be administered individually or in groups.

An advantage of the PMTO approach is that it teaches parents many of the foundational parenting strategies that are important for managing disruptive behavior (e.g., giving good commands, praising good behavior, using time-outs). It also includes problem-solving and communication training that can be helpful for addressing additional difficulties within the family unit that may reduce coercive processes over the long run. Thus, the main parenting strategies are encouragement, limit setting and discipline, effective monitoring/supervision, problem solving within the family context, and positive involvement within the family. There is ample evidence supporting the PMTO model as a strong intervention for promoting improvements in families (Forgatch & Patterson, 2010).

Helping the Noncompliant Child

Helping the Noncompliant Child (Forehand & Long, 2002; McMahon & Forehand, 2005) focuses explicitly on strategies that parents can use to promote appropriate behavior and reduce noncompliant behavior. Notably, the program is 5 weeks in length, making it an efficient approach to teaching parents effective child management strategies. Content covered within the program includes attending, rewarding, ignoring, giving directions, and time-out. As one of the pioneers of time-out from positive reinforcement for use with children with disruptive behavior disorders, Forehand provides a reliable source for parents.

Peed, Roberts, and Forehand (1977) reported on a trial where mothers were randomly assigned to receive the intervention or placed on a wait list. Families on the wait list received the treatment only after all measures were collected. Results of the study illustrated parents and children improved on measures in the clinic as well as in the home setting, whereas those in the wait-list group did not change. These findings support the effectiveness of this parenting program for youth with noncompliant and disruptive behaviors.

Summary of Evidence for Parent Training Interventions for Disruptive Behavior Disorders

As outlined above, there are a number of well-developed parent training programs available for caregivers of children with disruptive behavior disorders. The programs described are only a sampling of available resources. Additional parenting programs that are similar to the ones described above include the parent training program used by the Multimodal Treatment Study for ADHD (MTA; Wells et al., 2000), which further extend the evidence base for parenting programs for children with disruptive behavior disorders. For instance, the MTA parent training program, which includes many of the strategies developed within the parenting programs above and involves 35 sessions of group and/or individual parent training, resulted in positive outcomes on measures of parent–child interactions and parenting for parent training alone (MTA Cooperative Group, 1999; Wells et al., 2000) and when parent training was combined with medication management (Hinshaw et al., 2000; MTA Cooperative Group, 1999; Wells et al., 2006).

Thus, based on the available evidence, BPT is a clear evidence-based treatment for children with disruptive behavior disorders (see Evans et al., 2013; Eyberg et al., 2008; Pelham & Fabiano, 2008). BPT is a core component of a comprehensive approach to treatment for ADHD (Wells et al., 2000) as well as ODD/CD, and national organizations and practice parameters have identified BPT as an effective, first-line treatment (American Academy of Child and Adolescent Psychiatry, 1997; American Academy of Pediatrics, 2001; American Psychological Association Working Group on Psychoactive Medications for Children and Adolescents, 2006; Pelham & Fabiano, 2008). The preponderance of evidence thus suggests that efforts related to parent training should be redirected from debating the effectiveness of the intervention to disseminating, enhancing, and improving the use of behavioral interventions in community, school, and mental health settings. It is also worth noting that all the approaches described above are based on a generally consistent set of behavior modification principles. Below, a number of parameters of BPT that have been developed and researched are reviewed, followed by an overview of practical BPT strategies that can be utilized in practice.

FUTURE DIRECTIONS

Integrating BPT into a Chronic Model of Treatment

Because disruptive behavior disorders are typically chronic and persist through childhood into adolescence and adulthood, the integration of BPT into a chronic treatment model is needed. Currently, most parenting programs are self-contained packages that last from 2 to 4 months. A critical question relates to how follow-up of these programs should be conducted to promote maintenance of treatment gains and offer opportunities for additional BPT programming, as needed.

Current follow-up data suggest that the effects of BPT programs may persist years after the parenting program ends (Hood & Eyberg, 2003; MTA Cooperative Group, 2004; Reid et al., 2003; see expanded discussion of maintenance in Chapter 7). For instance, although the MTA study included a package of BPT, school-based interventions, and an intensive summer treatment program, the study provides interesting results related to the persistence of behavioral treatment effects. In the MTA study, children were randomly assigned to receive intensive behavior modification treatment, intensive medication management, the combination of both treatments, or assigned to a community control. At 14 months past baseline, combined and medication treatment conditions were generally reported to be superior to behavioral treatment alone and the community control (MTA Cooperative Group, 1999). However, at a 36-month assessment past baseline, none of the groups were significantly different from one another (Jensen et al., 2007). An inspection of mean scores indicates a gradual loss of treatment effects over time for the combination treatment and medication management group, and maintenance of treatment gains for the behavioral treatment and community control groups. Thus, similar to other studies, the MTA results suggest that behavioral treatment (that included an intensive BPT approach) was effective and persistent up to 2 years after the intensive treatment was faded.

Even though BPT effects appear to persist, it is also the case that a considerable portion of families treated with BPT will continue to struggle with child management and parenting issues after an initial course of treatment. For these families, there is little in the literature to guide the maintenance of treatment. One approach to promote maintenance in a chronic model of treatment is the use of booster sessions. Booster sessions are follow-up parent training meetings that occur on a less frequent basis after the initial course of BPT is completed. There is some evidence that booster sessions promote positive outcomes following BPT (McDonald & Budd, 1983), and though often included as a component in parent training programs, the effectiveness of booster sessions has received relatively little attention in the literature (Eyberg, Edwards, Boggs, & Foote, 1998).

An alternative to prescribed booster sessions following BPT is the Family Check-Up model (Stormshak & Dishion, 2002). In this model, an initial contact is made with a caregiver, a multimethod assessment is conducted (comparable to the approach described in Chapter 3), feedback from the assessment is provided, and then parents are offered a menu of potential strategies to use for intervention. The Family Check-Up can be conducted at regular intervals during targeted developmental transitions known to be difficult for children or adolescents with ADHD (e.g., entering kindergarten, middle school entry, obtaining a driver's license). A recent study used the Family Check-Up starting in sixth grade for children at risk for substance abuse; by ninth grade, families that received the Family Check-Up had parents who monitored their child better than those in a control condition, and had youths less likely to use alcohol, tobacco, and marijuana (Dishion, Nelson, & Kavanagh, 2003). This approach emphasizes family strengths, and it uses procedures known to enhance motivation to change, procedures that hold promise given potential difficulties in engaging parents of children with disruptive behavior disorders in BPT or maintenance programs.

Parametric Studies of BPT

The early BPT literature was notable in that it includes a number of sophisticated parametric studies of BPT components (e.g., time-out; see Hobbs & Forehand, 1977; MacDonough & Forehand, 1973). Although this work has continued, there have been fewer studies that investigate parameters of effective BPT programs more recently. For example, although most BPT programs introduce positive parenting strategies in sessions that precede those that address punishment strategies, there is only a single study that has investigated the order of parenting program session content, and this study suggested that the opposite order (i.e., punishment strategies taught first, followed by positive parenting strategies) was more effective and resulted in greater consumer satisfaction (Eisenstadt et al., 1993).

A number of parameters of BPT could use increased research attention for families with a child with ADHD. For instance, a critical question relates to psychosocial treatments combined with a BPT program. Some BPT programs include a concurrent child social skills building program (e.g., Cunningham et al., 1998; Pfiffner et al., 2007), whereas others include parent–child interactions as part of the intervention (e.g., PCIT). Miller and Prinz (2003) reported that no child involvement in treatment predicted termination from a parenting intervention—thus, these results suggest including a child component in BPT programming may be an important consideration to promote engagement, but it is an area in need of more study. Furthermore, many youth with behavioral challenges within the home setting have comparable challenges within other settings, such as school. Therefore school-related treatment is another important parameter to consider in effective BPT interventions (see Chapter 5). Due to this consideration, a number of studies have included a packaged treatment of parent and teacher interventions (e.g., Klein & Abikoff, 1997; MTA Cooperative Group, 1999). However, fewer studies have separated the home versus school treatment and compared these groups to a combined home and school condition (e.g., Barkley et al., 2000). Future studies that dismantle treatment packages that include BPT plus other intervention components are needed to determine the necessary and sufficient characteristics of a BPT intervention for youth with disruptive behavior disorders.

Additional parametric work is also needed to address the content of BPT programs. A traditional BPT program spans 8 to 12 weeks and introduces parenting topics sequentially, with approximately one new topic each week (see description of programs above). Other parenting programs may focus on a single problematic behavior (e.g., homework completion, peer relationship building) and introduce a number of strategies that are aimed at remediating that specific problem (e.g., Mikami, Lerner, Griggs, McGrath, & Calhoun, 2010; Power, Karustis, & Habboushe, 2001; Sanders, 1999; Zentall & Goldstein, 1999). It is currently unknown whether it is better to introduce parents to a group BPT program that introduces a number of parenting strategies in general, or to choose one problem and work with parents to introduce parenting strategies to address this primary reason for referral.

The frequency and number of sessions included in a parent training program is also an area in need of parametric study. Length of treatment has important implications, especially for a chronic and intensely impairing disorder such as ADHD. On the one hand, treatment needs to be sustained due to the severity of the problems associated with ADHD, but on the other hand, treatment cannot be so intensive or protracted that families become overwhelmed and drop out. In fact, one risk factor in the development of problematic child and adolescent behavior is that parents may become so taxed by the incredible demands that come with parenting a child with behavioral challenges that they "give up," resulting in less parental monitoring and inconsistent discipline, which will exacerbate negative outcomes (Dishion et al., 2004). Related to the discussion of booster sessions above, optimal strategies for structuring BPT programs to promote continued intervention efforts is an area in need of additional research.

The discussion above is by no means an exhaustive list of parameters in need of future study. Even basic questions such as whether parent training should be offered in groups versus individually, whether parent training takes place in a psychology clinic or an alternative location such as a home or school, and whether parent training should include parent–child interaction cannot be answered definitively by the current literature. Furthermore, how individual differences on the part of the child, parent, or family moderate these results is also an area in need of more study.

BPT Content May Need to Include Topics beyond Parenting Strategies

Parent factors (e.g., parental mental health) may be particularly important considerations in a BPT program. Reyno and McGrath (2006) conducted a meta-analysis of parent training outcome, and reported maternal psychopathology (e.g., depression) was significantly related to poor outcomes in BPT. Sonuga-Barke, Daley, and Thompson (2002) reported that the presence of maternal ADHD resulted in considerably less child improvement when compared to mothers without ADHD who participated in a BPT class. Thus, parent-focused interventions or sessions integrated into BPT to address these difficulties (e.g., anger management, organizational skills) may be needed. Perhaps because of these issues, BPT programs that permit discussions of potential issues beyond those explicitly related to parenting a child with a behavior problem promote persistence in treatment (Prinz & Miller, 1994).

Moreover, within the context of parent training, other evidence-based treatments might be employed. One example is the Coping with Depression Course (CWDC; Lewinsohn, Antonuccio, Steinmetz, & Teri, 1984). The CWDC is a 12-week, manualized, psychoeducational group treatment based on a social learning approach to depression. The CWDC emphasizes the relationship between thoughts, feelings, and behaviors to reduce negative affect and mood, and initial outcomes indicate this is a useful adjunct to, and perhaps enhances, standard BPT (Chronis, Gamble, Roberts, & Pelham, 2006). Evidence suggests that even traditional parent training programs, in which sessions focus only on parenting skills, have beneficial effects on marital satisfaction and maternal psychopathology even though these domains are not targeted directly (Anastopoulos, Shelton, DuPaul, & Guevremont, 1993; Pisterman et al., 1992), and it would be expected that directly intervening in these problem areas in conjunction with parent training would result in even larger improvement. Further study of the type of topics integrated, with whom, and to what degree or in what format is an area ripe for further investigation.

Dissemination of BPT

Behavioral interventions like those included in BPT programs are also interwoven into the fabric of society. Parents commonly use behavioral modification strategies with their children (e.g., time-out, grounding), and popular television shows illustrate the use of behavioral parenting strategies in homes (Sanders, Montgomery, & Brechman-Toussaint, 2000; *www. fox.com/nanny911; http://abc.go.com/primetime/supernanny*). Parent training programs also have been effectively integrated into parents' workplaces (Martin & Sanders, 2003), and parent training is used across the globe to effectively remediate problems related to disruptive behavior disorders (e.g., Dopfner et al., 2004).

Now that BPT is firmly established as an efficacious intervention, efforts to disseminate these effective strategies for treating disruptive behavior need to continue. Although BPT has been available for decades as an effective intervention, it is still not routinely available in clinical settings (Prinz & Sanders, 2007). Innovative, tiered models of parent training offerings, such as those available in the Triple-P Program, offer a promising means of reaching the greatest number of families that can benefit from the intervention (Sanders, 1999; Sanders & Turner, 2005). Efforts must continue to integrate BPT into school and community settings where families can access the programs with minimal disruption to family routines. Importantly, dissemination efforts must also continue to focus on strategies that will maintain the integrity of the BPT program once it is widely available in community settings. Approaches that bring parent training out of the clinic and into community situations such as the parents' workplace or the child's sports fields hold particular promise for engaging families (Fabiano et al., 2012; Martin & Sanders, 2003).

CONTENT OF BPT

In this section, specific strategies and skills are reviewed, and procedures for teaching parents how to use these skills are presented. These individual strategies are integrated into the packaged parent training programs described in the prior section of this chapter. Practitioners may find it useful to work with parents on a specific skill at times as well (e.g., a parent who is struggling with homework completion may find it useful to focus on establishing after-school routines; a teacher setting up a DRC may work with parents on establishing a home-based reward menu). A continued emphasis on function-based approaches to remediating disruptive behavior problems will be woven into the description of the specific parenting strategies.

Attending and Labeled Praise

As discussed in Chapter 1, children with disruptive behavior disorders receive a disproportionate amount of negative feedback, criticisms, reprimands, commands, and demands relative to typically developing children. For this reason, parenting intervention efforts usually start by encouraging parents to increase attention dedicated toward positive behaviors and begin to specifically compliment and praise the child for appropriate and prosocial behaviors. For all of the parenting programs reviewed above, these strategies are consistently emphasized early in the process. Interestingly, other interventions that aim at improving relationships, such as marital therapy, also emphasize positive communication and attention toward the other person as an important foundational skill (i.e., "listening and validation"; Gottman, Notarius, Gonso, & Markman, 1976; see also Chapter 5).

It is important for parents to understand that praise is both an antecedent to and a consequence for appropriate behavior. Thus, its role in a functional approach to intervention is to serve as both a precipitant of appropriate behavior and a consequence of it. Most parents can readily think of praise and attention as a consequence—if a child behaves appropriately, this positive attention can follow as a consequence. However, praise can also be an antecedent of behavior wherein the parent proactively attends to and praises the child, and this is where some behavioral change on the part of the parent may be necessary. This is because there is a common attitude toward parenting where we "let sleeping dogs lie"—if the child is behaving appropriately, most adults do not make an extra effort to "catch the child behaving." This is an efficient and practical way to parent if one is raising a typically developing child because there is not an overall negative context. Yet, if the child is receiving frequent negative feedback and more demands than would be expected, it is not hard to see how a child and parent can quickly fall into a pattern of misbehavior followed by reprimands, which would result in an overall net effect of negativity within the parent–child relationship. If the parent does not make a disciplined effort to observe, reinforce, and label appropriate behaviors, the family unit incorporates very little in the way of positive interaction. By proactively "catching the child behaving" a parent has the opportunity to use praise as an antecedent to future appropriate behaviors, as the child will be receiving attention for appropriate behaviors that the parent wants to increase.

Table 4.2 outlines some of the key components of effective praise and attending. Parents who utilize effective praise and attending will begin to attend to the child when he or she exhibits appropriate behaviors, even if they are minor appropriate behaviors (e.g., holding a door for the person next in line; flushing the toilet; putting the cap back on the salad dressing). The parent effectively using this strategy is essentially observing all child behavior and systematically attending to and providing labeled praise. Certain behaviors that are difficult for children with disruptive behavior disorders, such as complying with adult requests or commands, should receive praise every time they are exhibited (i.e., parents will

TABLE 4.2. Guidelines for Effective Praise and Attending

Specific component	Examples
Parent attends to the child when engaging in any appropriate behavior.	A parent who sees a child put his homework back in the backpack when finished without needing an instruction would say, "I am glad to see you being so responsible for your work." At dinnertime a parent might say, "I like how you are chewing with your mouth closed."
Parent follows any command with praise once compliance is attained.	After a child puts on her shoes when told, a parent would say, "Thank you for listening the first time." After being told to leave his little sister alone, a child does so, and the parent can state, "I appreciate how you stopped teasing once I asked you to."
Praise is labeled with the specific behavior that is being encouraged/targeted for increase.	"I like the way you used your walking feet in the store"; "Completing your chores before going outside was very mature of you"; "I am proud of the way you ignored that teasing on the bus." *Contrasting examples*: "Nice work"; "Good job"; "That was a good choice."
Labeled praise is paired with observable displays of encouragement, affection, enthusiasm, and attention.	Praise should include eye contact, an enthusiastic and positive tone of voice, smiling, and genuine content. It may include physical contact—pat on the back, ruffling hair, "high five"—as well as physical signs of approval such as a "thumbs up," "a-okay" sign.
Praise is provided at a rate more frequent than demands, reprimands, commands, and criticisms.	The rule of thumb is that the ratio of praise to reprimands should be offered at a ratio of at least three praise statements for every demand, reprimand, command, and criticism.
Praise is provided frequently for situations where the child is exhibiting fragile, emerging, or inconsistent appropriate behaviors.	A child who has difficulty inhibiting impulses to avoid interrupting two adults talking might initially receive attention and praise for appropriately waiting for a turn to talk after every sentence completed between the two adults. Persisting with an academic task such as homework may include praise and attending from the parent every minute (or less) initially, until the behavior of sustained attention becomes more consistent.
Praise occurs immediately, or as soon as is possible, following the behavior that is being encouraged.	Praise is immediate following compliance with a command. Praise is also provided immediately following other behaviors the parent wants to increase such as the use of good manners ("I like how you said please when you asked for a drink") and cooperating with peers ("I am impressed how you let your friend take the first turn on the video game").
Praise is balanced across everyone in the home.	Parents are mindful of providing praise equally across siblings. Parents use praise/compliments directed toward one another—for example: "Thanks for helping to unload the dishwasher; you know I don't like that job!"

provide praise for compliance *every* time the child follows through). A key component of effective praise is that it is labeled: the parent includes a comment that specifies the specific behavior for which the praise is being provided. This can be accomplished by starting statements with initial stems such as "I like how you . . . ," "I am proud of the way . . . ," and "That was really good to. . . ." These positive statements that list the specific behaviors that are the target of the positive attention help children to understand and identify the appropriate behaviors that are drawing the adult attention, so that they can repeat these behaviors that were the target of attention in the future.

Additional considerations in Table 4.2 relate to the "qualitative" aspects of praise and attending. For instance, the praise needs to be genuine. Children can readily see through a nongenuine approach, such as when a parent says "good job" with a disinterested look on his or her face. Nonlabeled praise can also be viewed as nongenuine. A bunch of "good jobs" in a row is not unlike a cashier saying "Have a nice day" to every person who checks out in a line—it is hard to maintain interest and engagement and to receive this message as a true affirmation. Sometimes parents "undo" praise as well. This can happen when a parent tags a negative at the end of a positive statement such as "I am glad you did your homework on time; why can't you do that every day?" or "I like the way you cooperated with your brother . . . it's a miracle." These negative, sarcastic, or critical comments paired with a praise statement not only devalue the praise, they also send the child a clear message of general disapproval and cynicism. To combat some of these aspects of praise that can undermine parental efforts, parents should focus on enthusiastically praising the child, using nonverbal social rewards (e.g., "thumbs-up") paired with verbal praise, and ensure that the praise is unencumbered by any negative connotation.

Rewards and Celebrations

It is stating the obvious to say people like rewards and celebrations. When the t-shirt cannon comes out at professional sporting events, everyone stands up and starts calling out for the free gift. We all enjoy a paycheck, which is a predictable reward for completing prescribed tasks at work. Rewards might also include special privileges or honors for meeting some benchmark or performing a specific behavior. For instance, our insurance rates might decrease if we are accident-free for 5 years. Children in a classroom who sit quietly and get their work done might earn a privilege such as taking a message down to the main office. People also like celebrations: we celebrate birthdays, anniversaries, births, retirements, and sometimes even Friday afternoons at the end of the work week. People feel special during these celebrations and they provide an opportunity to acknowledge progress. These rewards and celebrations are reinforcing because people value the social interactions and attention coupled within them, and they want to experience the positive and valuable experience again. Thus, they are an important component of interventions that aim to decrease problematic behaviors and increase positive and adaptive ones.

When supporting parents who are working with youth with disruptive behavior disorders, it is imperative to emphasize rewards and celebrations. One reason for this is that youth with disruptive behavior disorders appear to be hypersensitive to rewards, and he or she may persist in behaviors that are likely to result in the attainment of rewards (Byrd, Loeber, & Pardini, 2014). Thus, parents can capitalize on the focus of the youth by embedding rewards throughout daily activities. Furthermore, parents may find it preferable, and easier, to work with the child in a framework focused on earning positive consequences, rather than one focused on taking away privileges or enforcing negative consequences.

Before discussing the specifics of rewards, it is important to remark about a few questions parents often have when the issue of rewards is broached. First, some parents say they don't want to "bribe" their child for exhibiting appropriate behavior. It is important to distinguish the difference between a bribe and a reward. A bribe is when the reward is provided before the appropriate behavior to coax or coerce the outcome desired. The classic example is the shady businessman pushing the envelope of money across the table to a politician so he or she will vote in favor of the businessman's interests—this is not what is being advocated. In contrast, rewards occur only after the desired behavior is exhibited in a typical behavioral approach; the child has a choice to behave in a certain way to earn the contingent reward. Even if the reward is agreed upon ahead of time, it is only provided once behavioral expectations are met. Some parents also bristle at providing rewards for appropriate behavior. This ignores the obvious: most children are immersed in rewards all day (e.g., watching television, playing outdoors, access to snacks, using computers, access to toys, driving privileges). Parents who focus on rewards as part of a behavior management plan are not adding in *more* rewards. They are simply doing what the U.S. Army has done successfully in boot camps for decades: rights are first taken away and then they are earned back as privileges. Parents who do not think that children should be rewarded for doing the things they should do anyway (e.g., homework, chores, appropriate behavior) might be reminded that most *parents* go to work for their own reward that follows—a paycheck!

Table 4.3 lists some rewards that could be commonly employed for children with disruptive behavior disorders. Parents using reward programs can conceptualize some rewards as immediate and provided following a discrete target behavior. For example, a young child who follows the rule of "no screaming" during a trip to the grocery store might earn a quarter to use in the vending machine at the store exit or a teen who completes assigned homework may be provided a passcode to use the computer for a half-hour. Rewards may also be slightly delayed and provided following the child meeting daily goals (e.g., a positive report from school on a DRC; see Chapter 5). Finally, parents may choose to also include rewards that are earned after a longer demonstration of sustained, appropriate behavior (e.g., at the end of the week; after some criterion is attained such as 3 days in a row with no cursing).

Parents can be encouraged to be as creative as they want with rewards. For instance, my graduate advisor Bill Pelham gave good advice to me when I was working with parents who had a child who really wanted to earn a new video game. The parents felt that they would typically buy this video game for the child, but it was too much of a reward for only one day of good behavior. In this case, the child drew a picture of the cover of the video game, and the parents then cut the picture into 10 pieces. Each day the child met behavioral expectations he earned a piece and he glued it onto a piece of paper. Once all the pieces were earned he traded his picture in for the larger reward. The parents were satisfied that the child "truly" earned the reward, and the child enjoyed the process of marking his

TABLE 4.3. Examples of Rewards and Privileges

Category	Examples
Privileges	Extended bed time Outdoors time Chore pass Extended curfew Use of car/bike/rollerblades Phone Choose snack/meal/dessert
Screen time	Computer Television Tablet Phone
Tangibles	Money Snacks Toys/games/prizes
Adult attention	Special time with parent Choose an activity or game to play Call a parent or relative Read a book together
Long-term rewards	Toy/video game Playdate with a friend Sleepover with a friend Dinner at a restaurant Special activity (e.g., swimming or open gym, visiting a relative, going on a hike) Trip to arcade/bounce house/laser tag

progress. Another creative way to provide rewards is for parents to create a "grab bag" that includes a number of possible rewards (e.g., a get-out-of-chores free card, a card that says the parent will drive the child to school one morning, a dessert card) and the child chooses a random reward each time. This sort of approach can be further enhanced by adding one or two "big ticket" rewards to the grab bag (e.g., a $5 bill, a movie rental ticket). The child can be motivated by the randomness of the reward as well as the possibility of obtaining the large rewards.

Parents can often identify rewards by simply observing what their child chooses to do if he or she is given free access to activities and possessions in the home. This is a simple way to investigate the functional relationship between the child's behavior and rewards. If a child is frequently attempting to solicit parental attention (e.g., stating directly to a parent such things as "I'm bored," "Pay attention to me," or "Play with me"), then rewards related to adult attention may be most appropriate (i.e., they would meet the function of gaining attention). If a parent feels like he or she is constantly peeling his or her child away from a screen (e.g., computer, tablet, television), then screen time may be a good approach for rewards (i.e., it would meet the function of gaining a desired activity). Parents that find their child frequently requests new baseball cards, action figures, or makeup could use these items as rewards (i.e., it would meet the function of gaining tangibles).

Parents should also identify a variety of potential rewards so that they can construct reward menus. This prevents the child from becoming satiated quickly with the same reward. An example of this might be a child who is initially very motivated by access to video games, but once all the levels are successfully completed this reward may be less motivating for the child. One child who was in the clinic responding very well to television time as a reward began to exhibit an odd pattern where behavior deteriorated quite dramatically every Tuesday. We eventually learned that there was nothing on television the child liked to watch on Tuesday evenings. These examples illustrate the limits of using only single or relatively narrow rewards.

Celebrations should also be connected with reward programs. Celebrations are interwoven into the fabric of families—birthday cakes, artwork posted on the refrigerator, and cards in the mail are all components of celebrations that individuals find rewarding. As children with disruptive behavior disorders are working on improving their behavior, public displays and celebrations are an effective way to reinforce progress toward goals. Public posting is one approach to help parents celebrate and monitor progress. Public postings are also an effective way to motivate behavior as people enjoy having their good behavior publicized. Within communities public rewards include spotlights on the TV news or honor rolls in print, "Employee of the Month" postings within restaurants or stores, initials typed into an arcade game next to a high score, and students being placed on merit rolls in school for academic achievements. This same approach can be used by parents to celebrate good behavior within the home setting. Young children can place stickers on a "Merit Board" following appropriate behavior, parents can help elementary school students fill in a thermometer illustrating days without arguments over homework, and for teens appropriate behavior could be celebrated through a personal note in the lunchbox taken to school that day. Like the discussion of praise above, these celebrations need to be genuine and appropriate in frequency. Appropriately administered, they can serve as a good motivator for continued appropriate behavior.

Establishing Rules and Routines

Rules are all around us. Speed limit signs dot our roadways. The public pool rules remind us to avoid horseplay or gum chewing around the pool. Signs tell us to "Keep off the grass" or "Take a number and get in line." We are warned on the airplane not to disable a smoke alarm in the lavatory. Rules are even present in an office refrigerator—there may be a "Don't eat me" note stuck to someone's food he or she brought from home! Some rules are even presented without requiring the ability to read. For example, a picture of an index finger to the lips posted in the library or movie theater reminds us to remain silent. Simply defined, a rule is a regulation that defines appropriate conduct in or for a situation.

Rules are a cornerstone of parenting interventions. Although it might sound obvious that parents of children with disruptive behaviors should establish rules, families often have implicit rather than explicit rules and this is where difficulties emerge. For instance, an implicit rule within a family is that you behave at a relative's house when visiting. However, the definition of "behave" might be quite different depending on whether you ask the parent or the child. Because youth with disruptive behaviors receive so many messages about their behaviors from others, explicit rules are helpful for focusing on the main behavioral expectations that transcend specific situations. For children with disruptive behavior disorders, rules are also typically going to focus on the major behaviors that would result in immediate consequences if violated. Minor behaviors (e.g., completing chores, making eye contact) are best addressed through the use of effective commands as described below.

Examples of house rules include "No aggression," "Treat others with respect," "Use appropriate language," "Curfew is at 11:00 P.M.," "Listen to adult instructions the first time," "No cursing," "No friends allowed over without parent permission," "No alcohol or drugs," "Always tell the truth," "No stealing," and "Treat property with respect." Once a family establishes house rules, they should be clearly posted and continually reinforced. In much the same way parents label praise, corrective feedback about rule-following behaviors and rule violations should also be labeled (e.g., "You came home at 11:15 P.M., which breaks our rule of an 11:00 P.M. curfew"). Parents should also use the rules as antecedents to appropriate rule-following behavior. This can be done by reviewing the rules with the child or teen prior to each daily activity. Although at first this might seem like a lot of review, it is preferable to having to remind the child of the rules as a consequence after the violation has been exhibited.

Consistent routines are also a part of the structural antecedents that contribute to appropriate behavior. Predictability in daily activities helps children understand, anticipate, and prepare for transitions. If homework occurs every day at 3:30 P.M., and this has happened for months in a row, although homework is a nonpreferred activity, it will be hard to have a temper tantrum about it. In contrast, if homework occurs at inconsistent times, temper tantrums may seem like a reasonable strategy to attempt to defer homework to a later time. Routines also help parents keep organized, and this may be increasingly important as family schedules become busier. If a parent is able to stay organized, this should reduce overall levels of parental stress, which will allow the parent to dedicate more resources to his or her parenting.

Planned Ignoring

The importance of adult attention was highlighted within the prior discussion of praise and attending. Given that importance, attention can also be withheld to ensure this desired response is predominantly offered for appropriate rather than inappropriate behaviors. Recall the discussion within Chapter 1 of the typical morning within the life of a child with a disruptive behavior disorder. Nearly all the attention provided by adults, siblings, and peers was in response to a negative behavior, and very little attention was related to positive behaviors. Within this context, even the most conscientious parent providing labeled praise as much as possible would be fighting an uphill battle—the net amount of attention during the day is likely to remain directed toward negative behaviors. One way to address this issue is to simultaneously provide positive attention following appropriate behaviors and to strategically remove attention for negative behaviors, in particular the child's negative behaviors that have an express goal of gaining attention (e.g., complaining, interrupting).

A key issue with the strategy of planned ignoring relates to the behaviors that should or should not be ignored. A general rule of thumb is to ignore behaviors that are minor annoyances such as complaining, whining, fidgeting, crying, tattling, or throwing tantrums. The function of these behaviors is typically to obtain the adult's attention and get the adult involved in the situation either to remove a demand or limit or elicit one-on-one attention from the adult. By ignoring, the adult removes a potential reinforcer—negative reinforcement through the removal of a demand or positive reinforcement in the form of adult attention. There are many behaviors that should *not* be ignored and this includes any violation of house rules, aggression, disrespect, or any other behavior that an adult would not tolerate if it persists.

Parents can often find some increased motivation to use this strategy if they know ahead of time that children facing planned ignoring for a behavior often increase the frequency or intensity of that behavior before it decreases. This is known as an "extinction burst," and it is a fairly common behavioral pattern. Basically, behavior gets worse before it gets better. For instance, let's say a parent chooses to use planned ignoring for whining behavior at bedtime. Previously, the parent may have addressed the whining by telling the child to stop, negotiating with the child, or explaining why the bedtime was necessary. In an approach to addressing this behavior that includes planned ignoring whenever this demand is placed on the child, the parent would now focus only on issuing commands to go to bed, and avoid other discussions, corrective comments about the whining, or explanations. It is not hard to predict how the child may respond to this novel approach, as the demand of going to bed (one of the least fun activities in a child's entire day!) has not changed, only the parent's response to the child's protests has. A logical response from the child may be to guess that the parent simply did not hear the protests, or that they were not dramatic enough. Thus, the child could begin to protest in a louder or more annoying fashion. If the parent can maintain the planned ignoring approach, it would be likely that the child may increase the duration or intensity of the protests, but after some time (e.g., a week of bedtimes in a row) the child will learn that these protests are not useful in removing the demand. Coupled with a reward program that provides later bedtime for appropriate behavior, the parent can systematically teach the child that appropriate behavior is the means of having the demand modified. Thus, later bedtime is now achieved through appropriate behavior rather than inappropriate behavior.

A note on planned ignoring is important to mention. The extinction burst is a fairly reliable behavioral pattern for children when adults begin to ignore behaviors that previously worked to get adults to remove demands or focus attention on the child. There is a risk for parents of choosing to use planned ignoring if they are not willing to hold their ground and ignore through the expected increase in negative behavior. That is, that the child, if he or she is able to increase the negative behavior to a level that does elicit adult attention, may learn something the parent does not intend and may come to regret: namely, that the annoying behavior just needs to get *even worse* and then the parent will remove the demand or pay attention. This would set up the family for more severe and more frequent negative behavior in similar situations in the future. Thus, parents who choose to use planned ignoring must be willing to go "all in" in order to make the strategy work. It is during the time that the parent may be most inclined to attend to the child (i.e., when the behavior is most irritating) that the parent *must* ignore the behavior to prevent this situation from occurring.

Effective Commands, Requests, and Instructions

Forehand and his colleagues completed key work in the 1970s and 1980s when they systematically investigated parameters of commands and requests that either promoted or discouraged compliance. This work addressed the characteristics of one of the most common and important antecedents for child disruptive behavior: a parent command or demand. In these early studies, Forehand and his colleagues invited mothers into the laboratory with their young children. During these visits, Forehand asked the parents to request their child to behave in certain ways including picking up toys, completing tasks, and responding to other instructions. The research staff were positioned behind an observation window, and they recorded the instructions that occurred before compliance and noncompliance exhibited by the children. Sometimes the researchers instructed the mothers using a bug-in-the-ear device to observe child responses to specific commands or command sequences. The results of this program of research shed considerable light on oppositional behavior in young children. Results included that oppositional behavior increases as more commands are issued (Forehand & Scarboro, 1975), children comply more often to direct commands offered without any follow-up comments or reissued commands (Roberts, McMahon, Forehand, & Humphreys, 1978), and that vague, unclear, or poorly issued commands were a significant predictor of child noncompliance (Forehand, Wells, & Sturgis, 1978). These findings provided actionable suggestions for parents who issue many, many commands across a typical day.

Before discussing the characteristics of good commands, it is useful to review the characteristics of bad commands. These are well described in other sources (Forehand & Long, 2002; Pelham et al., 1998; Walker & Eaton-Walker, 1991). Table 4.4 lists some of the characteristics of inappropriate or poor commands.

One of the most obvious, yet important, characteristics of a poor command is issuing the command when the child is not attending. Anyone who has given an instruction to a spouse or partner dividing his or her attention between the instruction and the other task knows it is hard for an adult to attend to a command when simultaneously watching a television program or looking at the computer. It is therefore no surprise that this situation is also a challenge for a child. Poor commands are therefore those shouted from another room, issued in the presence of distractors, or issued when it is unclear whether the child is attending (e.g., the child is not making eye contact with the adult). Good commands are obtained only after attention is obtained. Sometimes this can be easily done by stating the child's name, pausing until the child looks at the adult, and then issuing the request. For

TABLE 4.4. Overview of Characteristics of Good Commands and Poor Commands

Inappropriate commands	Appropriate commands
• Issued when it is unclear whether the child is attending	• Issued once attention is obtained
• Contain multiple steps	• Issued in manageable steps
• Vague	• Specific
• Issued as a question	• Issued as a command/instruction
• Unclear phrasing ("Let's . . .")	• Clear phrasing
• Negatively phrased	• Positively phrased
• Wordy	• Precise
• Provide little time for compliance	• Provide adequate time for the child to comply (i.e., 5–10 seconds)
• Extended for a long period of time	• Limited to the present
• Repeated without consequences	• Followed by consequences for both compliance (e.g., praise) and noncompliance (e.g., repeat command)

Note. See Forehand and Long (2002), Pelham et al. (1998), and Walker and Eaton-Walker (1991).

very young children, a parent may need to get down on one knee, and tilt the child's chin up with the index finger to orient the child's eyes to the parent's own eyes. For older children a command to "look at me" may precede the main command. For teens, prompts such as "I am about to give an instruction" may help to orient the teen to the upcoming command. It should also be mentioned that although occasionally a call from the kitchen to come in for dinner will work for a hungry child, in most cases a parent needs to be physically in the same room when commands are issued to ensure that the child is attending.

Poor commands are also those that include a long list of behaviors linked together in a sequential order. Parents always groan when provided the example of, "Go to your room, put new pillowcases on the pillows, put the dirty laundry in the basket, take the basket out in the hall, pick up all the toys on the floor, set out your clothes for school tomorrow, and remember to put your library book in your backpack." Without fail a parent will exclaim, "I'd be lucky if my child did the first thing on that list." Many of the parents cannot even remember all the tasks within their own lengthy, chained command! Effective commands are issued one at a time. Following the appropriate completion of the initial request, parents should use this opportunity to praise the child for compliance, then issue the next command. At times it may be necessary for the parent to complete a task analysis to appropriately plan each step in the chain (e.g., outline all the steps needed to "clean the room" and issue each step in a logical, sequential order).

The next collection of poor command characteristics in Table 4.4 all relate to the phrasing of the command. Poor commands are vague, issued as questions, use unclear phrasing or are phrased in a negative way (i.e., tell what *not* to do), and are wordy. Vague commands are those many of us grew up with: "Pay attention," "Listen up," "Behave," "Zip it," "Knock it off," "Stop." These commands clearly imply some behavior that is to be exhibited, but from the point of view of a child they are not specific enough to inform the child of the behavior that would be compliant with the instruction. The positive way to phrase these commands would be to use specific language that outlines the behavioral expectation within the command. Rather than saying "Be good" to a fidgety child at a restaurant, which is vague, a parent could say "Sit on your bottom" which specifically describes the behavior that is requested. Another phrasing issue in commands relates to asking questions rather than stating a request. There is an inherent problem in commands phrased as questions ("Don't you think it's time to start your homework?"; "Won't you please put that down?"): they imply that the child has an option. Most situations where parents are issuing commands are not those where the child has a choice to comply or not. Therefore direct statements are more effective as they remove this false sense of optional compliance implied through question phrasing. Similar to commands phrased as questions, those that start with "Let's" are also problematic as they imply that the parent will be helping with the requested behavior ("let's" is short for "let us"). Unless a parent intends to sit down and assist with homework, the command "Let's get started with your homework" should be avoided. In addition to ensuring that instructions are direct, they should also be precise. Wordy commands such as "You know I love that table and you are making me really nervous with that drink you have because it is filled really high. Put it down, I don't want it to spill. It would kill me if it left a stain" include too much information for the teen to process. A better command would be "Take your drink into the kitchen." A final issue with the phrasing of commands relates to whether they are phrased positively or negatively. A negative command tells the child what *not* to do, rather than what to do. An example of this is readily apparent by watching a parent take a child to the grocery store. One using negative phrasing is faced with an unlimited number of behaviors that the child should not do ("Don't run," "Don't touch that," "Don't touch that either," "Don't pick that up, it's trash," "Don't stand in the middle of the aisle," etc.). A more efficient and effective manner of phrasing is to tell the child what he or she should do. For example, in the grocery store example, a parent may state, "Keep one hand on the shopping cart when we walk down this aisle."

Additional parameters of commands relate to the behaviors that surround or follow the command itself. These include how long compliance is expected for continuous behaviors, the amount of time required for compliance, and procedures that are established for dealing with noncompliance. Many parents, in a fit of frustration, have issued very poor commands such as "Don't ever talk to me like that again!" or "Look out the window and don't say a word for the rest of our car ride to Florida!" Commands that extend for a long period of time are doomed to fail. It is preferable for most children and teens to limit the command to a short period of time (e.g., "Sit at the table for the next 2 minutes"). Additionally, it is important that once a command is issued, the adult provides the child enough time to comply. Most parents expect instantaneous compliance with a request/command, and many will repeatedly issue a command in staccato fashion ("Come on get dressed, get going, get your clothes on, come on let's go . . .) in an effort to obtain this instant compliance. However, children often have to take time to process and follow the command. Broken down into its component parts, a child needs to receive the auditory stimuli that are part of the command, stop or inhibit the present behavior, hold the command in working memory as it is being processed, decide how to initiate the behavior, translate this cognition into a motor or verbal behavior, and then perform the behavior. This is actually a quite complex process, even for something as simple as getting dressed. Therefore good commands are typically followed by 5–10 seconds of silence prior to another verbalization by the parent. This provides the child with the space he or she needs to process and comply with the command. A final comment on commands will be addressed in the time-out section below: many poor commands are those that are repeated without consequences. A child told to go to bed 20 times before a parent gets angry and enforces this command with a threat of privilege removal will typically ignore the first 20 commands as they allow the parent to extend the bedtime. Good commands are always followed by an appropriate consequence; compliance is followed by praise and noncompliance is followed by a prearranged consequence that might include one more repetition of the command, time-out, or privilege removal.

Time-Out from Positive Reinforcement and Privilege Removal

Most parents will have to punish a child for misbehavior from time to time. A child with disruptive behaviors, by definition, will be exhibiting punishable behaviors much more frequently than a typical child. A common punishment procedure used for children is time-out from positive reinforcement, or time-out for short. Note that time-out is from positive reinforcement, which again reinforces the importance of the attending, rewards, and celebrations described above. Time-out will only be effective if implemented within the context of this overall positively reinforcing environment.

The principles of time-out have been used for generations. Essentially this is what the "dunce cap" in early schools was used for, and prison systems are based on a severe definition of time-out directed toward adults. One of the earliest academic descriptions of time-out came from A. W. Staats who wrote: "I extended those principles in originating the time-out procedure with my daughter when she was two. When she displayed inappropriate behavior I would pick her up and put her in her room in her crib and indicate she had to stay there until she stopped crying. If we were in a restaurant or other public place I would pick her up and go outside, without any rewarding social interaction" (*www2.hawaii. edu/~staats/contributions.htm*). Following this, innovators in the area of parent training for disruptive behavior included time-out within their programs. For instance, as part of parent management training, Patterson (1975a, p. 73) stated that time-out included a procedure wherein "the child is removed from the situation where he receives many reinforcers, and he is placed in a situation where he receives few, if any, reinforcers." Since that time, time-out has been widely disseminated as a behavioral management strategy for parents. Indeed, time-out is the most common recommendation by pediatricians for aggressive youth (Scholer, Nix, & Patterson, 2006). Furthermore, consistent with the description in Chapter 1 of the considerably greater demands placed on parents of children with disruptive behaviors, mothers of children with ADHD administer more time-outs than mothers of typically developing youth (Stormont-Spurgin & Zentall, 2006). Time-out has thus been around for a long time and it is one of the most prominent success stories for the dissemination of behavioral interventions from the laboratory to applied settings.

Unfortunately, along with the widespread dissemination has come some drift from the initial behavioral principles that made time-out such a powerful tool. Time-out is one of the most common behavioral interventions that parents say "doesn't work." Barkin, Scheindlin, Ip, Richardson, and Finch (2007) report that up to a third of parents report their approach to disciplining their child is not effective. These outcomes should not be too surprising—parents have to enact punishments such as time-out in challenging situations such as a house rule violation or aggressive behavior. These situations can be emotionally charged for both the child and the parent, and this may be one reason why procedures are not implemented consistently or drift may occur. Few of us are at our best when preoccupied by the emotions of anger, sadness, or embarrassment. Thus, some principles are important to keep in mind prior to the need to implement a punishment procedure such as time-out.

One important consideration is a reminder that time-out will only work if it is time-out from positive reinforcement. When parents report using time-out for misbehavior during homework, chores, at bedtime, or before the school bus is arriving, it is questionable whether these activities are positively reinforcing and whether time-out is an effective strategy. Other activities may be more or less reinforcing, depending on the child. Although many children find swimming to be very reinforcing, I can recall a child I worked with who exhibited an aggressive act every time he entered the pool area to elicit the assignment of a time-out. It turns out this child was afraid of swimming and engaged in the negative behavior to purposely receive a time-out and avoid the feared situation. In this situation time-out *was* the reinforcing situation! Parents must also ensure that time-outs are truly nonreinforcing. Sending a child to her room for time-out is likely to be ineffective if the room includes a computer, a television, toys, and/or a cellphone. Finally, if a parent finds him- or herself repeatedly administering time-outs, multiple times a day, the procedure is somehow breaking down. One way for a parent to know the time-out approach is working is that time-outs are assigned only infrequently. This means that the overall environment is positively reinforcing and the time-out approach is serving as a deterrent to negative behaviors because the child wants to remain in the reinforcing environment. An exception to this situation is that when time-outs are first implemented, the child's behavior may get worse before it gets better due to an extinction burst.

When deciding how to implement a time-out, parents should consider a number of parameters that go into the time-out plan. Table 4.5 lists these parameters and some of the evidence for particular approaches (Hobbs & Forehand, 1977; MacDonough & Forehand, 1973). Some initial parameters of time-out that parents must consider include how to administer the time-out when it is appropriate to do so. This involves some preplanning to decide on behaviors that will result in time-outs, how the child will be informed of the time-out, where the time-out will occur, how long it will last, and how it will end. Each of these considerations is now briefly reviewed.

Times outs should be administered in a matter-of-fact way. Presumably if yelling, lecturing, scolding, mean faces, and wagging fingers worked, there would be no reason to implement time-out in the first place as most children with disruptive behavior challenges have experienced all these consequences multiple times. Parents should establish rules for time-out that include the rule violations that result in time-out (e.g., aggression, repeatedly

TABLE 4.5. Parameters of Time-Out from Positive Reinforcement to Be Addressed in Intervention Planning

Parameter	Recommendations from research evidence
Providing an explanation of the reason for time-out	No clear evidence this makes a difference with respect to child behavior but it may help parents to be consistent in implementation by making them verbally state the reason for time-out.
Providing a warning prior to time-out	Warnings may reduce the need for time-outs because they serve as an antecedent to behavior change. This is most appropriate for noncompliant behavior and less appropriate for aggressive/destructive behavior.
Location of time-out	There is not much evidence to support isolation versus observation. Permitting the child to observe "time-in" may have some benefit as it permits the child to see what is being missed while in time-out.
Duration of time-out	In general, shorter time-outs (e.g., 5 minutes) are preferable to longer time-outs (e.g., 30 minutes).
Release contingencies	Release contingent on some duration of appropriate behavior during time-out appears prudent. There is some evidence this improves behavior within a time-out.

Note. See Fabiano et al. (2004); Hobbs and Forehand (1977); MacDonough and Forehand (1973); Roberts (1982); and Scarboro and Forehand (1975).

not listening to instructions) and for within the time-out (e.g., exhibit no further rule breaking or disrespectful behavior, stay in the time-out location until released). Parents should also establish a time-out area. This might be a consistent area such as the back step or in the corner of the dining room in a specific chair. Alternatively, parents can define time-out areas depending on the physical location of the child and family (e.g., outdoors, in a public place like a store, in the kitchen). An additional consideration prior to assigning time-outs is the appropriate duration of the time-out. There is some diversity within recommendations within the field for appropriate lengths of time-out, but the available evidence generally shows time-outs do not have to be lengthy to be effective. A study by Fabiano and colleagues (2004) with youth with ADHD had both short (5 minutes) and long (15 minutes) time-outs and the shorter version appeared to work comparably to the longer version. Similar findings wherein shorter time-outs were generally equivalent to longer versions were reported for studies with noncompliant youth (Hobbs & Forehand, 1977). Because monitoring a time-out is stressful for the parent and unpleasant for the child, a shorter version should be used if it is relatively equivalent to the longer form. Furthermore, this puts the child back into time-in sooner, promoting opportunities for the child to receive praise, rewards, and build competencies in functional areas. Release from time-out is another issue that should be decided in advance. There is not a large amount of evidence to guide parents on the best approach for releasing a child from time-out, but it seems prudent to require a short duration of calm and rule-following behavior prior to ending the time-out. To forego this expectation might result in the child engaging in another behavior at the release that would simply result in another time-out. Once the time-out is over, the parent may have a brief interaction with the child to ask him or her what resulted in the time-out to ensure the child understands the reason for the punishment. Past that, the motivation of the parent should be to reengage the child within the time-in environment as quickly as possible. Admittedly, this might be difficult if the child engaged in a behavior that made the parent angry and resulted in the initial time-out, but in the long run this contrast between time-out and time-in is critical if time-out is eventually going to serve the purpose of suppressing negative behavior because it is an aversive situation relative to time-in.

Time-outs in a physical location become less prudent for teenagers, and in this case grounding can serve as a mechanism to time the teen out from positive reinforcement. For instance, the parent can take away the car, cell phone, access to friends, or other privileges. Although the inclination may be to remove these privileges for long periods of time (e.g., weeks or school marking periods), this is not advised. Indeed, parents would have a hard time maintaining such punishments consistently for long periods of time; the longer away the punishment is from the precipitating event, the harder it is for the teen to make the connection between the problematic behavior and the punishment (eventually it will just seem unfair), and perhaps most importantly if the parent takes away reinforcers for long periods of time the punishment is no longer time-out from positive reinforcement as there is no opportunity to experience time-in. Thus, it is generally recommended that punishments last no longer than a day or two for older teens unless the infraction is a grievous one (e.g., breaking the law).

Planning Ahead

Antecedents and consequences can provide strong influences on behaviors. Parents who are working on modifying and manipulating antecedents are typically on higher ground than those who are consistently working on consequences. This is because consequences are typically implemented after a negative behavior has already occurred, and few children or parents are at their best following a negative behavior. On the contrary, if a parent can prevent a negative behavior from occurring, the parent is able to avoid the unpleasantness that surrounds a negative behavior and subsequent punishments, and instead can enjoy the time with the child when appropriate behavior is exhibited.

Thus, planning ahead is an important parenting strategy. Some of the planning ahead principles are also embedded within the prior discussion of routines. Parents can also plan ahead to capitalize on their child's own preferences and behaviors. One way to do this is to use Premack principles throughout a daily schedule. Put simply, the Premack principle orders activities such that a less preferable activity occurs prior to a more preferable activity. This might include such approaches as "When you eat your vegetables, then you can have dessert," "When you complete your chores, then you can go outside," or "When you are done with your homework, then you can read your book from the library." This strategy works because a motivating activity is put right after the less motivating activity. This is also one reason we do not receive paychecks on Mondays: paychecks are only distributed at the end of the week after one's work is completed.

Parents may also find it helpful to plan ahead when routines or schedules may change. Children with disruptive behavior disorders may have difficulty negotiating the less predictable and at times overstimulating situations such as visits to a relative's home, going to the store or a restaurant, or beginning a new recreational or community activity. In these situations, parents can use the strategies outlined above to create new rules, contingencies, rewards, and reasonable punishments to inform the child or teen of expectations ahead of time, which may serve to prevent any difficulties from occurring. If the child does exhibit challenging behaviors, there is also no question about how to proceed, as this plan was already created and reviewed.

SUMMARY

In this chapter, packaged parenting programs were reviewed. These are often an efficient and effective way to introduce the foundational parenting strategies discussed in the latter half of the chapter. Figure 4.1 outlines an approach to working with parents that emphasizes

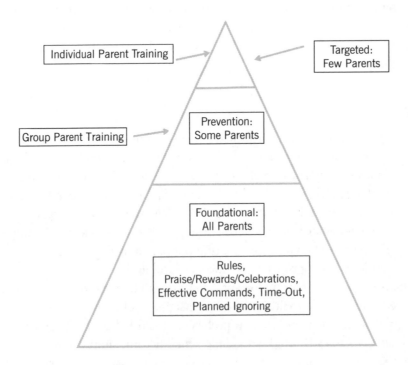

FIGURE 4.1. Organizational structure of interventions within a tiered approach to behavior management skill building with parents.

the establishment of foundational strategies for all parents. Many parents of youth with disruptive behavior disorders will find it necessary to also participate in group parent training classes to provide the opportunity to develop and try out these skills over a dedicated period of time. Fewer parents may need individual parent training, and this is represented by the top of the pyramid in the figure. Practitioners working with parents may find it helpful to discuss and facilitate the use of these foundational strategies in tandem with the school-based and skills-based strategies discussed in Chapters 5 and 6.

CHAPTER 5

School Interventions

Disruptive behavior disorders are a prevalent issue within school settings across developmental levels. Teachers consistently identify effective classroom management as one of the predominant, if not the most important, issues facing them within their professional practice (Rose & Gallup, 2006). Anyone who has tried to manage a group of 25 youth and direct them all toward a unified set of behavioral goals knows that this can be a difficult charge. Furthermore, any large group of youth is likely to be populated with some individuals who exhibit greater rates of disruptive behaviors, which will increase the overall levels of disruption within the classroom. Given this situation, it is surprising that teachers receive relatively little formal instruction and applied practice within teacher education programs on effective classroom management procedures, and once teachers begin working in classrooms the support is even less because the emphasis is typically on effective instruction and curricula implementation. Yet, teachers will have considerable difficulty teaching if they cannot organize, reinforce, and provide corrective feedback to their students in an effective and ongoing manner.

Similar to the discussion within Chapter 4, it is important to acknowledge that teachers are likely to be engaging in many activities to manage and corral disruptive behavior within the classroom. The issue is that for youth with significant levels of disruptive behaviors, some of these strategies may be insufficient, or even counterproductive at times. The same coercive process described within Chapter 1 can also be developed within the classroom context with teachers. It is not hard to imagine how a child could begin with mild, disruptive behaviors such as calling out, eye rolling and complaining, or passive noncompliance when the teacher gives instructions, and the teacher responds to these behaviors with reprimands, looks of disapproval, and public corrective feedback. Over time, this kind of interaction can evolve into more direct disruptive behaviors from the child such as talking back, verbally abusive comments, or active noncompliance (e.g., pushing away an uncompleted seatwork assignment). These negative behaviors are likely to result in even more intensive teacher efforts to control the child's behavior, which may include yelling, removal of privileges, and ignoring of inappropriate behaviors albeit in a nonsystematic manner. Eventually, the child may greatly increase the intensity of disruptive behavior (e.g., pushing the entire desk over when the teacher instructs the student to begin seatwork; exhibiting serious disrespect through cursing or yelling at the teacher). It is important to note that in this situation, the child and the teacher did not begin at the most intensive level of behavioral excess and efforts to control it: this was a process that evolved across time. This indicates that it is also a process that can be rectified through a careful and systematic approach to reverse some of the escalating negative behaviors on the part of the child and the teacher.

Within this chapter, procedures are reviewed for managing disruptive behavior and promoting appropriate behavior across levels of intensity. Initial strategies will be those teachers can use for a whole class or within a whole school. Additional strategies will be of a more targeted nature that is more appropriate for children with greater levels of disruptive behavior. Chapter 10 includes some additional discussion of how all these interventions might be integrated across a tiered, problem-solving approach to managing behavior within school settings. For the purposes of this chapter, the strategies will be organized first into foundational level approaches, second, into those that can be used to prevent more serious disruptive behaviors, and finally strategies that can be used in schools for youth with serious and ongoing challenges with disruptive behavior. Figure 5.1 illustrates how these levels/tiers of intervention are organized across the school and classroom in a widely accepted prevention/intervention framework. The reader is referred to a number of other excellent resources for promoting appropriate behavior and reducing disruptive behaviors in class-

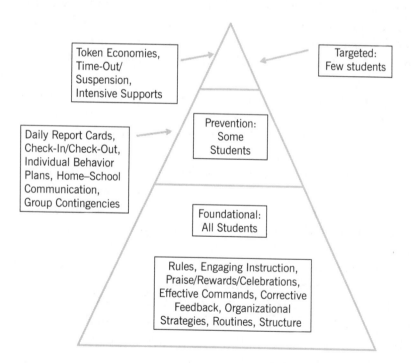

FIGURE 5.1. Organizational structure of interventions within a tiered approach to behavior management in schools.

rooms (e.g., DuPaul & Stoner, 2004; Gresham, 2015; Lane et al., 2011; Walker, Colvin, & Ramsey, 1994).

FOUNDATIONAL STRATEGIES

As noted in Chapter 1, children with disruptive behavior disorders experience considerable negative experiences throughout a typical school day. These include reprimands, commands, redirections, and ignoring of appropriate behaviors. These negative experiences can be from teachers, peers, and other school staff such as bus drivers, aides, office and cafeteria staff, and administrators. To counteract this negativity, there are a number of strategies that should be implemented within classrooms in a universal way to ensure a reinforcing, supportive, and consistent environment for the child. Many of these strategies were introduced within Chapter 4 in the discussion of effective parenting strategies. Therefore, the discussion in the present chapter will be tailored to school situations rather than repeating information already reviewed within the context of the home and in parenting.

School and Classroom Rules

Rules within schools are ubiquitous. There are rules for the hallway (e.g., "Use an inside voice," "Walk at all times"), rules for the classroom (e.g., "Be respectful of one another," "Listen to directions," "Do your best work"), rules for the cafeteria ("Remain in your seat," "Use appropriate table manners"), rules for the bus (e.g., "Stay seated at all times while the bus is in motion"), and rules for the playground ("Be safe"). These rules are often posted prominently for all to see and they set the tone for the expectations within certain school settings.

It is important to acknowledge that while rules are important antecedents to appropriate behavior and provide a clear set of expectations for students, rules alone are unlikely to provide sufficient incentive for promoting appropriate behaviors in classroom settings. An early study by Madsen, Becker, and Thomas (1968) illustrated that the implementation of rules alone in a classroom did not result in appreciable changes in student behavior. It was only when the rules were combined with other interventions (e.g., systematic praise for appropriate behavior and ignoring inappropriate behavior) that the rules were effective. Thus, additional interventions to combine with clear school/classroom rules are described in the sections that follow.

Rules are useful within schools, however, given that students come from various home situations and parental expectations. Within this diversity of experience, school rules serve to level the playing field by orienting all students to the expectations within the school building and associated areas (e.g., the bus). Teachers should routinely review rules before every activity (e.g., "We are going into the hall; remember, our rules are 'No talking,' 'Stay in a single-file line to the right,' and 'Walk at all times.'"). As students become more familiar with rules, teachers can ask the children to provide an overview of the rules to check for their memory of specific rules in specific situations. Although it may seem redundant at times, it is likely best to review the rules prior to every activity throughout the school year. This serves as an antecedent to the children's appropriate behavior. Roadway rules illustrate this point: speed limit signs are not posted for the first month or two of the year and then taken down with the expectation that all drivers will continue to follow the speed limit. Certainly, new drivers would be at a disadvantage because they would not even know there was an expectation for a limit on speed, and some drivers familiar with the road would be unlikely to remember the specific expectation for that roadway. Even drivers who are on the road everyday will see the sign and slow down appropriately due to the prompt because they may be distracted by other things and not focused on the behavior of keeping their speed within the limit. School rules are much the same: they should be prominently posted throughout the year, regularly reviewed, and used to orient and clarify behavioral expectations for students throughout the school grounds.

Rules are also very important within middle and high schools, perhaps even more important because multiple adults interact with students during the day. This means that rules not only need to be clearly conveyed to the children and teens, modifications also need to be clearly specified. In a high school, for example, it may be allowable to move around the room in a science lab, but this would not be allowed in a language arts seminar. Efforts to make rules consistent across the school are advisable for some behaviors including rules regarding eating and drinking, cell phone use, being on time and prepared for class, expectations for behavior in the hallway (e.g., appropriate voice level, stay to the right on a stairwell whether going up or down), bullying, and inappropriate language. If teachers are inconsistent in their attention to particular rules, this could serve to undermine the efforts of other teachers. Schoolwide committees with representation from each grade level and/or subject area may be one vehicle for effectively identifying key school rules to be emphasized across school areas and classrooms. Table 5.1 lists some examples of school rules across settings and grade levels.

Praise, Compliments, and Celebrations

Chapter 4 outlined some of the basic principles of praise and compliments. Praise should be liberally integrated into school settings. One of the tenets within Chapter 4 was that praise should be issued more frequently in situations where someone is learning a new skill or behavior. This is a fundamental activity within school settings, where children are continually learning new skills! There are multiple targets of praise that include academic, socioemotional, adult and peer interaction, behavioral, and social skills. Adults can praise the occurrence of the behaviors that support and facilitate the acquisition and development of targeted competencies. This public praise also serves to cue students to the important behaviors they should be working to develop, and it sets a positive tone and climate for the classroom.

However, in spite of the rationale for embedding praise throughout school activities, there is clear evidence that praise happens infrequently within schools, and rates decrease precipitously as students progress through school (Brophy & Good, 1986). Specifically, White (1975) illustrated how teachers frequently used praise in kindergarten and first grade,

TABLE 5.1. Examples of School Rules across Settings and Grade Levels

Setting	Elementary school	Middle school	High school
Classroom	"Be respectful of others." "Follow adult instructions." "Use materials appropriately." "Keep hands and feet to yourself." "Use an 'inside voice.'" "Raise your hand to talk." "Stay in your seat or area." "Try your best." "Complete your work."	"Arrive on time for class." "Arrive prepared for class." "Raise your hand to contribute or ask for help."	"Arrive on time for class." "Arrive prepared for class." "Contribute to class discussions." "No cell phones or earbuds allowed." "No food or drink allowed." "Respect adults and peers."
Hallway	"Use an 'inside voice'/ Remain quiet." "Walk at all times." "Remain in a single-file line." "Keep hands and feet to yourself."	"Travel only to/from your locker." "Travel to necessary areas only." "Walk at all times." "No cell phone use." "Keep hands and feet to yourself."	"Walk at all times." "Use appropriate language." "Use an appropriate voice level." "Remain to the right side when traveling."
Cafeteria	"Use appropriate table manners." "Stay in your assigned seat." "Ask for permission to get up." "Use an 'inside voice.'" "Treat others with respect."	"Use appropriate table manners." "Treat others with respect." "Listen to adult directions."	"Use appropriate table manners." "Treat others with respect." "Remain within your designated area."
Bus	"Remain in your seat." "Use an appropriate voice level." "Treat others respectfully." "Listen to the busdriver."	"Remain in your seat." "Use an appropriate voice level." "Treat others respectfully." "Listen to the bus driver."	"Remain in your seat." "Use an appropriate voice level." "Treat others respectfully." "Listen to the bus driver."
School Grounds	"Remain in your assigned area." "Treat property with care and respect." "Listen to adult instructions."	"No cell phones allowed during school hours." "No smoking/drinking/ drugs."	"No smoking/drinking/ drugs." "Appropriate attire is required at all times."

Note. These represent only a sampling of rules for these settings and grade levels. Schools may find additional rules are appropriate for their setting and student body. Rules should be positively phrased when possible (i.e., tell the student what to do), and they should be reviewed prior to beginning each new activity.

but their use of praise decreased with every successive grade level. One might speculate on the reasons for this decrease, and there are likely to be multiple contributors. First, adults might think that praise is only to be used for young children, and that older children do not need it. This cannot be true: even most adults appreciate a compliment or an acknowledgment for a job well done. There would not be a greeting card section for thank-you notes if older individuals were unappreciative of acknowledgements. Second, perhaps children just become less responsive to praise. Yet, this is also unlikely, as many interventions that employ praise work with children beyond kindergarten and first grade (e.g., Fabiano et al., 2007). Third, perhaps as children get older and progress through school, educational systems become more outcomes-oriented (e.g., demonstrating proficiency on statewide tests) and less process-oriented. Regardless of the reason, this drop in praise over time within school settings is one of the most readily addressable, low-cost, and potentially effective situations that can be targeted in efforts to promote appropriate behavior within school settings.

Celebrations are also embedded within the fabric of schools. These include handing out cupcakes for a birthday, morning announcements that identify students on a sports team by name, and earning honor/merit roll status. The problem with these celebrations is that that they are either noncontingent on behavior (e.g., a birthday) or so infrequent that they do not serve as a consistent motivator (e.g., quarterly merit roll announcements). Educators could better leverage school celebrations to better support the behavior of youth who have trouble following rules in school. This could be done by making celebrations contingent on behavioral outcomes, and the celebrations do not even have to be elaborate ones. This is illustrated in a study conducted with grade-school children in a cafeteria (Fabiano et al., 2008). In this study, children were provided feedback on their behavior during the cafeteria period, and they earned tickets based on their behavior that went into a drawing for a class-wide prize. This initial intervention improved behavior, but the school discipline committee wanted to improve behavior even more. It was determined that the top three classes that had the most tickets earned for good behavior each week, regardless of whether they earned a reward in the ticket drawing, would earn a banner placed over their door that proclaimed their excellent behavior. The school staff from the principal to the custodians made a point to visit those classrooms and reinforce the good behavior through compliments directed toward the class. Following the implementation of this intervention, behavior improved by an additional 40%. This is a remarkable outcome given that the public posting of the honor and extra effort by school staff to praise and attend to it was the only program modification needed.

School-Based Rewards

Related to praise is another type of reinforcement: tangible rewards and privileges. Schools are embedded with all kinds of privileges and rewards, but just as in the home, as pointed out in the discussion in Chapter 4, these potential powerful reinforcers are usually not offered contingent on student behavior. Teachers could think carefully about the activities, privileges, and tangibles that students talk about, work for, or ask for, and access to these could easily be made contingent on appropriate behavior.

Teachers in elementary school could walk around their classroom and create a list of potential rewards. These include activities such as computer time, free reading, free time, and games. Also included are tangibles such as edibles, stickers, school supplies such as pencils or special erasers, and prizes. Some rewards could be negative reinforcers that allow the student to avoid something he or she dislikes. Examples of this would be a "get out of homework" pass or an early ending to a lesson or seatwork assignment. Rewards can also include privileges. Anyone who has ever been in an elementary school knows that the line leader is a coveted place, as is a teacher's helper or office messenger. These roles can be made into privileges. Additional privileges might include special accommodations. For instance, a student might be allowed to complete an assignment of their choice on a colored piece of paper, use a special pencil or pen to write it, or sit anywhere in the room of their choosing to listen to a teacher lecture.

Opportunities to Respond

One of the strongest contributors to positive academic outcomes is how often teachers provide opportunities for students to provide academic responses as well as behavioral responses. Response opportunities represent chances for the student or students to provide answers, apply concepts or new information, or contribute to group discussions on class content. Research has highlighted the fact that the number of academic response opportunities present in the classroom is related to student learning and appropriate behavior within schools (e.g., Sutherland & Wehby, 2001).

The "traditional" classroom might be characterized as one with few opportunities to respond. Consider a class where the teacher asks students to open their reading book to a particular page and students take turns reading one paragraph at a time, beginning with the first student in the first row and cycling through all the students in the room after that. This is a reasonably organized way to read through the material, but it is woefully lacking in response opportunities because only one child reads aloud at a time. Some students may not attend to the material until they hear the child next to them begin reading, and then they will find their place and attend for only a short part of the lesson. This inefficient approach can be contrasted with innovative approaches that greatly increase academic response opportunities including peer-tutoring interventions (Fuchs & Fuchs, 1997). In a classwide peer-tutoring intervention, children are paired with a classmate, and they work together to complete a reading, math, or other academic assignment. During the paired activity one of the two partners is reading or completing an academic activity while the other partner closely supervises and supports the completion of the task. From a response opportunity perspective, the students are completing many more academic responses compared to the traditional approach described. Words read in the traditional approach might number 100 whereas in the peer-tutoring approach the words read may be in the thousands. Across multiple classes and an entire school year it is not hard to understand the advantage of this approach. Outcome data also support it, with youth participating within peer tutoring in classrooms improving in academic as well as social outcomes (Fuchs & Fuchs, 1997).

Increased opportunities to make academic responses in the classroom have also improved the behavior of youth with disruptive behavior disorders, in particular (Sutherland & Wehby, 2001). In these studies, children with disruptive behavior were observed to be on task at a greater rate and to improve their academic achievement. To realize the positive effects of the provision of opportunities to make academic responses, researchers suggest that there should be three to four of these opportunities, on average, per minute (Englert, 1983; Stichter et al., 2009). In addition to providing these opportunities to respond, teachers must also offer time for students to think about and process academic material rather than forging ahead (Stichter et al., 2009). Unfortunately, the Sutherland and Wehby (2001) review reported generally low rates of opportunities to make academic responses within the classrooms of youth with disruptive behaviors. Thus, this approach is one that teachers could work to integrate within classrooms immediately, and it should promote improved behavior and academic productivity on the part of students.

Effective and Engaging Activity Planning

Parents of children with ADHD often remark that their child, who has attention difficulties when confronted with homework, chores, or other boring tasks, can "sit through an entire movie" or "play video games for hours." This does not mean that the child has a lack of attention problems, but rather it highlights how context and situation can serve as an antecedent to particular behaviors. Educators who are confronted with teaching challenging subjects or dry material can likely attest to the difficulty of maintaining student attention and persistence with the task relative to other subjects or topics of greater interest. This is one reason why educators often strive to be highly creative in their lesson planning to ensure interest even when the topic might not lend itself to what the child would choose to do if left to do so on his or her own.

Planning ahead within the construction of class activities is one way teachers can choose to manage classroom behaviors using an antecedent control strategy. This is clearly apparent if one considers "downtime" within classrooms. Transitions, wait time, free periods, standing around in line, and sitting quietly until the final student completes a task or activity are all low-stimulation situations within classrooms. As such, these are potential antecedents to negative or disruptive behaviors because if the child is not engaged with something proactive and positive, he or she may decide to engage in a behavior that is negative.

Classroom planning begins with routines and schedules. Educators that run their class with a consistent schedule use antecedent control to their advantage. Children's knowledge of the current activity, how much time will be allotted to the activity, and which activity will come next can promote engagement with the activity. Indeed, over time children may begin to run the schedule themselves as they get used to the predictability of the daily activities. If one thinks schedules are not important to children, one has to simply go to a kindergarten class on the first day of school: teachers spend the entire day answering questions such as

"When do I get to go home?"; "When is lunch?"; "Can we play with the toys?" A predictable schedule offsets the need for these questions and likely also promotes a feeling of calm and security among the children who can reliably know what activity will be coming next.

Once a teacher has a schedule planned, the schedule must be executed. That means that activities need to start and end on time. One of the ways this can be promoted is to budget the time needed for transitioning into schedules. For example, a morning schedule might include bellwork, English/language arts, math, physical education, and science. Educators can enhance this schedule by planning ahead to think about how much time is required for each of these activities, and also plan for the time needed to transition in and out of the activities. Furthermore, within activities, time can be budgeted to ensure that children are spending most of their time in learning activities rather than moving from one activity to another or in instructions. Figure 5.2 illustrates an overall morning schedule. Note that the times for specific activities are fixed, but each is further broken down to allot an appropriate amount of time for transitions, cleanup, instruction, and learning activities. Teachers who plan ahead should not go over the time provided, in general. For instance, a teacher who was adhering to the schedule would know that she spent too much time on instruction if there was not enough time for the children to begin the worksheets.

Effective Commands and Requests

Teachers have to give a considerable number of instructions throughout the school day. Chapter 4 provides an outline of instructions that are good versus poor in wording and presentation, so they will not be repeated here (see Table 4.4 for more information). Rather, strategies educators can use to focus on enhancing their use of effective commands and requests will be emphasized.

To illustrate how many commands occur in a typical school day, a recent study by Reddy, Fabiano, Dudek, and Hsu (2013) provides some foundational information. In this study, observers watched 317 elementary school teachers across grades kindergarten to fifth during two half-hour observation periods, representing two different academic lessons. During these observations, teachers provided an average of approximately 20 commands. Eighty-five percent of these commands were rated as being well constructed, with 15% of the commands rated as "vague." Using this estimate of 20 commands in a half-hour, and estimating that approximately 6 hours are spent in the teacher's classroom, this yields 240 commands per day. Extrapolating outward, that is 1,200 commands issued by the teacher each week, and across 40 weeks of a school year that is nearly 50,000 commands! Importantly, this is only an estimate, with some teachers likely issuing many more commands based on their classroom demands, grade level, or personal instructional style (e.g., the range for commands in Reddy et al., 2013, included an upper bound of 51 per observation period). These commands represent opportunities to comply with and exhibit productive behavior, but it is important to note that each of these almost 50,000 commands also represents opportunities for noncompliance, one of the most significant disruptive behaviors within educational settings.

Time	Activity	Time Breakdown
8:00–8:20 A.M.	Bellwork	8:00–8:15: bellwork 8:15–8:20: reminder to finish work and turn it in
8:20–8:25 A.M.	Inform children that bellwork time is over Take attendance Transition to next activity	
8:25–9:55 A.M.	English/language arts	8:25–8:45: small groups Session 1* 8:45–9:05: small groups Session 2* 9:05–9:25: small groups Session 3* 9:25–9:50: large-group instruction 9:50–9:55: clean up materials and return to seat
9:55–10:00 A.M.	Transition to math Get up and stretch	
10:00–10:45 A.M.	Math class	10:00–10:10: flash card "Around the World Game" 10:10–10:15: review of content from prior class 10:15–10:20: partner review worksheet 10:20–10:30: large-group instruction 10:30–10:40: begin to practice; remainder of worksheet for homework 10:40–10:45: clean up and line up for specials
10:45–11:30 A.M.	Physical education	10:45–10:50: change to gym clothes 10:50–10:55: warm-up 10:55–11:15: badminton 11:15–11:20: free play 11:20–11:30: change clothes and line up
11:30 A.M.–12:00 P.M.	Lunch	

FIGURE 5.2. Example of a morning school schedule. *Children are divided into small groups by skill level in English/language arts. Children rotate through three stations: (1) teacher-led small group; (2) independent worksheet calibrated to group reading level; (3) peer partner reading exercise.

Starting with the knowledge of an estimated 50,000 commands per year, teachers can improve their practice by making their overall number of commands more efficient and effective. The first way to do this is to be mindful of the commands that are issued and determine whether some commands need to be issued at all. As discussed, routines, rules, and schedules can help promote behavioral activation within students, and if the students are complying on their own, and a command does not need to be issued, this removes an opportunity in the classroom for noncompliance. To the extent that a command is also demanding and unpleasant for a child, it also removes a negative stimulus from the classroom. Furthermore, Reddy and colleagues (2013) provided an estimate of 15% of commands being poorly worded, issued as questions rather than statements or including a long chain of expected behaviors, all characteristics of commands that make it more difficult for the child

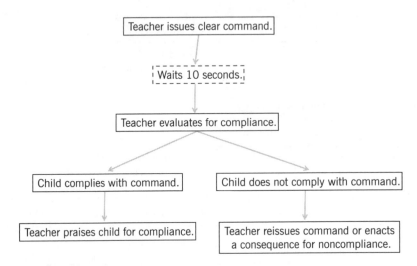

FIGURE 5.3. Flowchart illustrating how a teacher should issue commands and evaluate compliance. See Pelham et al. (1998) and Walker and Eaton-Walker (1991) for expanded discussion.

to understand behavioral expectation and therefore comply. This means that approximately 7,500 commands in a given year are of the types that yield a low probability of compliance. If teachers could simply reduce the commands that have a low probability for compliance, either by issuing clearer commands or forgoing a command in that instance altogether, a significant amount of noncompliance within classrooms might be reduced.

Corrective Feedback

Feedback is a core component of learning and instruction. Feedback is also a core aspect of behavior management. This starts from early in development when children learn the word "no" and feedback continues as children progress throughout development. Corrective feedback can be helpful in scaffolding children toward exhibiting appropriate behaviors more consistently, and it also provides a model for other children to observe and learn about appropriate behavior indirectly.

Appropriate components of corrective feedback are not unlike the guidelines for effective praise. It must be labeled in a manner to describe exactly what behavior was problematic. It must be genuine and supportive—that is, provided in a manner that tells the child what went wrong but also how to exhibit a more appropriate behavior or make a better choice in the future. Corrective feedback should avoid relying on "don't," "stop," or "no" statements, but rather label the behavior and provide a reason why it is problematic followed by a positive behavioral suggestion. If a child is running down the hall, rather than shouting, "Don't run in the hallway!" an effective corrective feedback statement might be a calm reminder like, "Running is not allowed in the hall. Walk at all times." Feedback must occur frequently when a child is working to master a new skill or behavior, and should be faded as children become more proficient. Finally, the frequency of corrective feedback must be appropriately balanced with labeled praise using the "three praise statements for every negative statement" rule of thumb. This means that if corrective feedback is issued more frequently when a child is learning a new skill, then the educator will need to also issue much more praise during this time to keep the three-to-one ratio of praise to negative statements balanced.

Discussion of Foundational Strategies

There are some issues with respect to the implementation of school behavioral management principles that should be discussed. First, there is a robust trend within schools that the use of positive strategies such as praise and rewards decreases precipitously from the early primary grades to very minimal use by the later primary grades into middle and high school. This is noted by teachers, students, and objective observations (e.g., Lewis, 2001; White, 1975). Second, when considering interventions used to manage behavior, attention is often directed toward youth who are exhibiting negative behaviors rather than what is often the majority of youth who are behaving appropriately. Finally, it is also the case that these strategies need to be maintained over a long period of time (i.e., an entire school year or school years), and this is something difficult to do outside a systematic classwide or schoolwide framework. For this reason, such frameworks, populated with these foundational strategies that are implemented universally, have found support within educational settings.

Examples of these behavioral support frameworks include PBIS (Sugai et al., 1999), RTI approaches that use behavior management strategies (Vujnovic et al., 2014), and other systematic behavior management frameworks (Pelham et al., 2005). A discussion of how such frameworks can be effectively implemented to help youth with disruptive behavior disorders occurs within Chapter 10.

As a final note, it is important to emphasize that if an educator, classroom, and/or school is not sufficiently or effectively implementing foundational strategies, this should be corrected before moving to institute the more intensive interventions that follow as prevention or targeted strategies. The foundational strategies provide the bedrock upon which more intensive strategies should be instituted. Fabiano and colleagues (2007) illustrated how the removal of praise, effective commands, rewards, and effective consequences can result in large decrements in appropriate classroom behavior. In this study, a classroom without typical foundation supports was created in an experimental situation. Children with ADHD attended each classroom and rates of rule violations within the classrooms without effective foundational strategies averaged 1.5 rule violations, per child, per minute within a 30-minute seatwork class period. It is not hard to extrapolate this rate of rule violations across an entire school day, week, and year, and to consider the negative impact on student, teacher, and classroom functioning. It is further easy to underscore how *stressful* this situation would be for an educator and other students. Thus, the use of foundational strategies can reduce overall levels of disruption to make efforts to implement more intensive interventions more useful.

PREVENTION STRATEGIES

The foundational strategies described above should be used liberally with all students throughout the school year. For the ensuing discussions of prevention and targeted strategies, it is presumed that these foundational strategies are being implemented, and that the implementation is being done with integrity and fidelity. If that is not the case, it is recommended that efforts be made to improve the foundational strategies prior to the implementation of more intensive interventions.

Daily Report Cards

DRCs have long been used within school settings to manage and reduce disruptive behaviors (Kelley, 1990; Volpe & Fabiano, 2012). The DRC is an operationalized list of a child's target behaviors (e.g., interrupting, noncompliance, low academic productivity), and includes specific criteria for meeting each behavioral goal (e.g., interrupts *three* or fewer times during math instruction). Teachers provide immediate feedback to the child regarding target behaviors on the DRC. The DRC is sent home with the child each day, and parents provide home-based privileges (e.g., use of bicycle, computer time) contingent on meeting DRC goals. Thus, the home and school are linked on a daily basis, a critical aspect of coordination across settings.

The DRC has long been used effectively to treat disruptive behavior, monitor outcomes, and open a daily line of communication between teachers and the child's parents (DuPaul & Eckert, 1997; DuPaul & Stoner, 2004; Kelley, 1990; O'Leary & Pelham, 1978; O'Leary et al., 1976; Pelham et al., 1998, 2005; Pfiffner et al., 2007, 2013; Sheridan & Kratochwill, 2008; Vannest, Davis, Davis, Mason, & Burke, 2010; Volpe & Fabiano, 2012), and it is a procedure aligned with a long tradition of using contingency management with children with disruptive behavior in general educational settings (e.g., Hops & Walker, 1988; Hops et al., 2013) and in special education settings (Reid, Maag, Vasa, & Wright, 1994; Schnoes et al., 2006; Vannest et al., 2010).

Used on an ongoing basis, the DRC offers multiple advantages to educators in schools. It is sensitive to environmental modifications, and it is also a useful device for communicating with parents regarding the child's behavior in school. Teacher feedback to the child regarding progress toward goals and explicit feedback regarding whether goals are met may also serve as an antecedent to future appropriate behavior (Sugai & Colvin, 1997), and contribute to amenable parent–teacher relationships. Thus, in addition to immediate behavioral effects, the DRC may be used as a data-driven monitoring device for schools to use to evaluate the progress of children in special education programs on a daily basis.

In its simplest form, a DRC is a list of behavioral goals that are well defined and stated in a way that the teacher can evaluate quickly and easily whether the goal was met. This evaluation then is shared with the child after each evaluation point. The DRC is then returned home with the child, and it is shared with the parents. Parents provide prearranged rewards/privileges for goal attainment at home each evening. These components together comprise the DRC intervention. It is important to note that any one of the components alone may be used, but it is only when they are all used together in concert that the DRC intervention is being used.

There are a number of resources that can be used to develop a DRC. Websites include guides (see *http://ccf.buffalo.edu/pdf/school_daily_report_card.pdf*) and DRC generators (see *http://interventioncentral.org/teacher-resources/behavior-rating-scales-report-card-maker*). Individuals interested in more extensive descriptions of how to construct and implement DRCs are guided to helpful publications (e.g., Kelley, 1990; Volpe & Fabiano, 2013).

To create a DRC, educators must first identify and operationalize targeted behaviors to include academic behaviors (e.g., "Completes assignment within time given"; "Returns completed homework with 80% accuracy"; "Prepared for call with all required materials"), adult-directed behaviors (e.g., "No instances of disrespectful language directed toward an adult"; "Complies with adult requests the first time"; "Accepts adult feedback without any instances of arguing"), peer-directed behaviors (e.g., "No more than three instances of teasing"; "No reports of bullying"), or other behaviors (e.g., "No more than two interruptions during the class discussion"; "Arrives on time for class"). Generally, no more than three to five targets are listed on the DRC. Next, the teacher determines when the targets should be evaluated: morning/afternoon, once a day, or after each subject/lesson. One important step in a DRC construction is the specification of criteria for meeting the goal. This includes stating "no more than two reminders for interruptions" rather than a general goal of "works quietly." The criterion for each goal is important, as this helps the child keep track of his or her behavior and also encourages the teacher to be precise with the feedback provided.

Form 5.1 at the end of the chapter provides an example of a DRC that might be suitable for use in elementary school settings. Form 5.2 illustrates a DRC that might be appropriate for a middle or high school student. In both cases, the principles behind the DRC are identical: the child/teen has clearly defined targeted behaviors, there is a criterion for each behavior (e.g., "three or fewer instances"; "no instances") that clearly identifies how many instances are able to be exhibited prior to missing the target, and there are home rewards that are provided to the child/teen contingent on meeting goals throughout the day.

Figure 5.4 illustrates potential home rewards that can be used. Home rewards for the most part should be those that are naturally occurring. A good way to think about home rewards for a DRC is to use a similar principle to that used in the U.S. Army: things that are commonly expected as rights are taken away and instead provided to the child contingently as a privilege based on appropriate behavioral expectations that are met. Rewards are only limited by the parent's creativity. In past clinical work, rewards including walking down the road to watch construction vehicles after school, use of a special mechanical pencil for homework, sleeping in a pop-up tent rather than the bed, and completing a science project with a parent. There are always the usual suspects for rewards/privileges as well, including screen time (computer, tablet, television, video game console), access to a phone, staying up past bedtime, having a friend over/playing outside, and snacks/desserts.

For many children with disruptive behavior disorders, school rewards may also be needed for DRCs, as the latency between the behavioral feedback and the reward may be too great for some children, especially those with more frequent behavioral challenges or greater impulsivity. In these cases, rewards could be generated in the same way as they are

Percentage of Goals Met	Rewards
10–50%	30 minutes of television before bed OR Dessert OR Call Grandma
51–75%	**Choose 2:** 30 minutes of television before bed Watch cartoon on computer Dessert 1 baseball card Extra story Stay up 15 extra minutes
75–99%	**Choose 3:** 30 minutes of television before bed Watch cartoon on computer Dessert 1 baseball card Extra story Stay up 15 extra minutes
100%	Special walk around the block in the dark with flashlights OR Choose snack from special grabbag for tomorrow's lunch

FIGURE 5.4. Example of a home reward plan for a DRC.

for the home—an educator can think about what the child chooses to do at school (go on the computer, play with friends, play with the class pet, listen to headphones, homework pass) and access to these rewards could be made contingent on meeting DRC goals as well. An additional in-school enhancement is to add a check-in–check-out procedure. This is a formal approach wherein a teacher, school counselor, or other school professional meets with the child each morning. After a warm, genuine greeting, the child turns in the signed DRC from the day before, has the behavioral goals and rewards reviewed, and receives positive encouragement about meeting goals during the day. At the end of the day, the child returns to this individual, reviews the results recorded on the DRC, and receives praise or encouragement as appropriate. This approach has been shown to support behavioral improvements within elementary school settings (Todd, Campbell, Meyer, & Horner, 2008).

Supplementing daily home rewards and possibly any school-based rewards would be weekly rewards. These are typically longer-term rewards of higher value. For instance, some children may wish to have playdates with peers or relatives, rent a movie or video game, or go to a park. These rewards are often impractical for daily provision, but they may be feasible for weekends. Parents can establish expectations that promote sustained, appropriate behavior (e.g., at least four out of five DRCs within a school week that earn 80% of targeted goals), and provide the larger, weekly rewards contingent on meeting the long-term goal. Notably, the daily rewards are continued regardless of progress toward the weekly goal to ensure the child has appropriate motivation to strive toward exhibiting appropriate behavior each day.

Behavioral Contracts

Behavioral contracts are a useful approach for dealing with disruptive behavior within educational settings. Many of the same principles of the DRC described above are embedded within an approach that uses a behavioral contract. Differences are that the behavioral contract may focus on behaviors that occur at a lower base rate than those targeted on a DRC. Whereas a DRC may target behaviors such as interruptions, talking back, or seatwork completion, which can occur frequently, a behavioral contract may focus on truancy, fighting, stealing, or insubordination, which may occur less often (if they are occurring often, then a DRC may be a more appropriate strategy to implement).

A behavioral contract is straightforward—it operationally defines the target behavior, and it outlines the consequences for meeting or not meeting the behavioral goal. Behavioral contracts may also outline the individuals responsible for implementing each part of the contract, how progress will be assessed and monitored, and contracts will also typically include a date upon which the contract will be reevaluated. Form 5.3 at the end of this chapter provides an example of a behavioral contract template that might be utilized. This approach to preventive intervention may be best utilized in middle and high schools where children may be capable of being more mindful of their behavior and long-term goals.

An important component of the behavior contract is that it explicitly includes the child/teen within the discussion of the targeted behavior, its operalization, and the consequences for meeting or not meeting the goals. This format of intervention may be more important as children become adolescents and are expected to take a greater role in self-management. Furthermore, the process of conducting a meeting and discussion to establish a behavioral contract also helps engage the child prior to the next occurrence of the problem behavior in a proactive manner. The establishment of clear expectations and predetermined consequences could serve to act as an antecedent to future appropriate behavior for the child. The act of signing the paper also makes the expectations and contingencies "official" such that the child/teen knows exactly what to expect. As a side effect, the signed document may also promote consistent implementation of the consequences (both positive and negative) on the part of the adults because the signed contract becomes the binding approach agreed upon by all parties.

Function-Based Approaches

Children who exhibit disruptive behavior disorders within classroom settings may do so because the behaviors viewed as negative by teachers, parents, or peers result in some functional benefit for the child. These functional benefits might not always be obvious or consistent with the point of view of educators of other children within the class. For instance, a child may tantrum whenever it is time to go out to the recess playground, resulting in the child being sent to the disciplinarian's office and consequently missing out on recess time. Most children are enthusiastic about heading out to the playground for recess, so this behavior may seem on its face to be puzzling. However, if a teacher discovers that the child is being bullied or teased within the context of recess, this behavior becomes more sensible from the child's perspective as it allows the child to avoid a situation that is unpleasant. From the child's point of view, avoiding unpleasant recess interactions is more rewarding than the fun activities embedded within recess, making this tantrum functionally useful because it permits the child to avoid a situation that is disliked.

A comparable situation arises often within the context of academic tasks in schools. Few children are enthusiastic about completing academic seatwork, sitting through a lesson, or engaging in other school-related tasks. This is because these academic situations are demanding—the child must focus attention and sustain it, use multiple cognitive strategies alone and in concert, and often also engage in other behaviors that are demanding such as handwriting, peer interactions, maintaining information within working memory, and working under time pressure. Tantrums in this case are also functionally useful as they may permit the child to avoid an unpleasant task.

Escape/Avoidance

For children exhibiting disruptive behaviors to escape/avoid a situation they dislike, multiple functional approaches can be utilized. One is the Premack approach that puts less desirable activities prior to more desirable activities. The child can be instructed that "When you complete your math worksheet, then you can read the book you chose in the library." Or the teacher could state, "When you complete the partner think–pair–share assignment, then you can have free time." These "When . . . then . . ." statements help reduce the value of avoidance because they promote the value of completing the less preferable task by highlighting the more preferable activity to follow.

Another way to deal with escape/avoidance-maintained behaviors is to provide socially appropriate mechanisms for the child to use to escape an undesired activity. For example, a child could be provided with three red cards at the beginning of the school day or class period. Each red card could permit the child to sit out an activity for 2 minutes, regardless of the ongoing situation. The child would agree to use the cards rather than acting out. The knowledge that there was a means of escaping the activity could serve as an antecedent to more appropriate behavior on the part of the child as the need to exhibit negative behaviors to escape become less needed.

A final way to deal with negative behaviors used to escape/avoid an activity is to use a postponed time-out intervention. In this approach, the educator determines which activities the child enjoys and finds rewarding (e.g., free time, recess, specials). The child is then informed that each minute of an undesired activity that is missed due to negative behaviors (e.g., temper tantrums) will be deducted from the desired activity the next time the desired activity occurs. In this way, the child will lose a desired activity from the efforts to escape an undesired activity. This approach could be further enhanced by having the child complete the undesired activity during the time he or she is sitting out of the rewarding activity (e.g., uncompleted seatwork that the child refused to complete during academic instruction time could be given to the child to complete as he or she sits out recess), making it less likely they will engage in behaviors to escape or avoid the undesirable activity in the future.

Gain to Self—Tangible

Sometimes a child may exhibit disruptive behavior to gain a tangible item. This functional behavior may occur within peer interactions. For instance, a child may walk up to a peer and snatch a marker that is being used because she may want to use it herself. This type of behavior may also occur on a playground where a child takes a kickball away from a group of children playing an organized game because he wants to bounce the ball himself. Sometimes a child may engage in stealing behavior in order to gain money, objects, or other possessions.

If the function of the behavior is to obtain a tangible item for the self, educators can use an intervention approach that integrates this function into the plan. The DRC is a formal way to provide tangible rewards for appropriate behavior. Teachers could institute an intervention plan that uses similar principles, but on a less formal basis. For instance, young children might earn stickers for completing an assignment within the time given. Children may also earn access to art supplies or recess toys following the display of appropriate social interaction behaviors in the classroom or on the playground. If children are exhibiting stealing behaviors, an educator may develop socially appropriate ways for the child to gain tangibles. For instance, if a child was stealing money from other kids to buy snacks in the cafeteria, a behavioral program might be instituted wherein the student could earn points toward a free snack certificate based on appropriate classroom behavior (after making restitution for the stolen money).

Attention

A teacher's attention is one of the most sought-after rewards within school settings. One only has to observe what happens when a teacher provides individual attention to a student or even a visitor to the classroom; more times than not, children will come up with reasons to interrupt or solicit the teacher's attention (sometimes by breaking a classroom rule, which is often a highly effective way to get the teacher to pay attention to the rule-breaker). Similar to the discussion about parents in Chapter 4, therefore, a teacher can systematically use attention to shape and encourage appropriate behavior and discourage inappropriate behavior.

Many teachers naturally use their attention to influence student behavior. For example, when leading a group lesson, a teacher may ask a question and only call on students raising their hands. A teacher may even remark, "I am looking to call on students with their hands raised quietly." By only calling on students with quietly raised hands, the teacher encourages this behavior. By simultaneously ignoring children who call out or who raise their hands and also shout "Ooh, ooh, ooh!" as they lean forward across the desk, the teacher ensures attention is only provided for the positive behavior and over time it will encourage quietly raised hands within the classroom.

Attention can be a very powerful tool for educators for reducing disruptive behavior, if the function of the child's inappropriate behavior is to gain attention. Take the results of a study conducted by Pinkston, Reese, LeBlanc, and Baer (1973). An active preschooler was observed to attack other students unprovoked, exhibit aggression toward staff (biting, scratching), and directing verbally abusive statements toward others. During baseline, teachers were asked to respond to the negative behaviors as they typically would; their responses included verbal corrective feedback, explanations for why the behavior was inappropriate, and other verbal and nonverbal attention directed to the child following an aggressive or negative behavior. During the intervention phase of this study, teachers were instructed to change the way they provided attention during one of the child's negative behavior episodes. Rather than attending to the child, they immediately directed their attention to the victim of the negative behavior. For example, if the child was aggressive toward a classmate, rather than reprimanding the child for the negative behavior, they immediately directed sympathetic attention toward the classmate, and tried to console the classmate (e.g., "I am proud of you for ignoring that hitting; here, let's go play with this toy car together"). Teachers also directed positive attention toward the target child when he was exhibiting positive behaviors that were cooperative and that followed classroom rules. Results for this intervention approach, that *only included the systematic redirecting of teacher attention*, indicated immediate and sustained improvement in the problem child's appropriate behavior. He averaged approximately 25% of peer interactions engaging in aggressive behavior during the baseline and reversal conditions, and this dropped dramatically during intervention conditions. The positive results were also maintained, with the child only exhibiting aggressive behavior during 3% of peer interactions during a 1-month follow-up observation.

This study is a terrific example of how teachers can use their attention alone to modify and maintain the rate of appropriate behavior exhibited in the classroom. Clearly, one function of the study child's aggressive and verbally abusive behavior was to gain attention, as the behaviors decreased as soon as they no longer gained adult or peer attention. Conversely, it also illustrates how teacher attention may indirectly or perhaps in some cases directly serve to maintain disruptive and aggressive behavior within educational settings. Teachers who want to promote appropriate behavior can use their attention to encourage students to follow rules and function effectively within group settings.

Skill Deficit

Although not technically a function, at times a child may exhibit an inappropriate behavior due to a skills deficit. This could be, for example, a learning disability, some limits in organizational ability, or social skills deficits. These skills deficits may serve as antecedents for negative behaviors that permit the child to gain attention (e.g., by poking or teasing) or escape a task (e.g., by exhibiting noncompliant behavior). Thus, the functional relationship between the problem behavior and the antecedent factor can be potentially remediated by improving competencies and skills. For instance, a child who frequently teases another child to gain attention could be taught how to become more proficient in a sports activity children in the class enjoy playing in order to integrate the child into a peer setting in an appropriate manner. Peer attention can then be obtained through prosocial participation in the activity rather than through the negative behavior of teasing. Additional details on skill-building interventions are discussed in Chapter 6.

Group Contingencies

Prevention strategies may also include whole-classroom interventions. There are a number of whole-class interventions that can be used to target overall levels of classroom disruptive behavior, or that might be focused on a single student or handful of students. These classwide interventions are often part of group contingency programs, within which consequences apply to the whole group. There are three main types of group contingencies: (1) interdependent, (2) dependent, and (3) independent (Maggin, Johnson, Chafouleas, Ruberto, & Berggren, 2012). An interdependent group contingency provides a reinforcer to the entire class based on overall group functioning. For instance, the class might earn a pizza party if there are fewer than 10 behavioral referrals from the bus within a month. A dependent group contingency provides a group with a consequence if a single student or small group of students meets a goal. For instance, the entire class might earn extra free time if there are no reports of Stephen bullying other kids that day. Finally, an independent group contingency sets a behavioral goal for the class, but each student who meets the goal can earn the reward regardless of the functioning of other students or the whole group. In this case, each student who avoids a behavioral write-up for inappropriate behavior within the cafeteria between Monday and Thursday can attend a "special" lunch in the classroom with the teacher on Friday. Maggin and colleagues (2012) reported that the most common group contingency within the behavioral treatment literature was a program wherein consequences were provided to the entire class based on whole-class behavior.

Group contingencies are effective interventions for promoting appropriate behavior if the educator determines that the problem is classwide and not the result of an individual student or small group of students. In the latter case, the individual approaches described above are recommended. Group contingencies are also effective if peer attention is a current maintainer of inappropriate behavior. For instance, children "clowning around" may elicit giggles, smiles, and encouragement to misbehave from other classmates who have nothing to lose. However, if the students are invested in exhibiting appropriate behavior because it results in a reward, those "clowning" behaviors are no longer funny—they become an irritant because they may impede access to a reward. Thus, group contingencies are a potential way to rapidly modify the peer ecology in the classroom such that negative behaviors no longer elicit positive peer attention. Group contingencies are often useful in situations where peer attention is maintaining inappropriate behaviors and/or adult supervision is low. Anyone who has ever ridden a school bus knows that the prior sentence accurately describes that peer context! Greene, Bailey, and Barber (1981) illustrated how group contingencies can reduce disruptive behavior on a bus. In this example, an automated sound device recorded whether noise levels exceeded a prearranged threshold, as well as the duration of the loud noise. For the middle school students on the bus, a light panel at the front of the bus "lit up" when the noise level was exceeded. The middle schoolers on the bus could listen to music as long as they did not exceed the noise level threshold more than a prearranged number of times. This simple intervention, which required no additional staff, significantly improved student behavior using the group contingency. Teachers can institute group contingencies such as these through a discussion with the class where they identify the group issue or problem (e.g., tattling, cheating), determine the threshold for meeting the group goal (e.g., "No more than five instances of tattling per day"; "No one caught cheating during the day"), and then list positive (5 minutes of free time for the whole class at 2:25 P.M.) and negative (no free time for anyone in the class) consequences for meeting or not meeting the group goal. Form 5.4 at the end of this chapter can be used to create a group contingency program with the class.

A prominent and successful example of a group contingency aimed at reducing disruptive behavior is the Good Behavior Game (GBG; Barrish, Saunders, & Wolf, 1969; Embry, 2002). The GBG was developed as a way to control disruptive behavior in a whole class. The GBG requires no additional supplies or materials, can be implemented after minimal training for teachers and students, and leverages current resources in the classroom to effectively reduce disruptive behavior.

An educator can establish the GBG in a classroom by dividing the students into teams. This can be done by grouping students in "islands" of desks, designating each row as a team, or by some other means of linking students together. Then, the teacher identifies a target behavior or group of target behaviors (i.e., interruptions in class; teasing peers; getting out of seat without permission). Next, children are instructed that each time the target behavior occurs, the team will receive a mark on the whiteboard in a small square designated for the team. Teams that have fewer than a predetermined number of marks (e.g., five), or the team that has the fewest marks if greater than five, earns a reward. In the Barrish and colleagues (1969) paper rewards included the privilege of wearing a "victory tag" around the neck so the winners could be easily identified in the classroom, a star was put next to the students' names on the winner chart, the students on the winning team lined up first for lunch, and the winning team could take part in a 30-minute free time at the end of the day. Students who were on a team that had more than five marks and/or did not win the competition did not earn the privileges and continued to complete schoolwork during the 30-minute free-time period. Contemporary iterations of the GBG institute rewards after each activity to reduce the wait time for team rewards. Furthermore, the current versions of the GBG emphasize teams earning the reward if they meet a particular threshold of good behavior (i.e., "No more than 10 instances of the target behavior during English/language arts class instruction"). This reduces the competition between teams and fosters cooperation within teams. Few teachers would complain if all students earned the rewards because this would mean the behavior in the class was good throughout the lesson!

The GBG is elegant in its simplicity. The peer ecology is instantly changed by putting children together on teams and making rewards contingent on team success, as it now encourages children themselves to promote good behavior among their team members. Interruptions that were funny or mimicked by other children prior to the GBG are met by cold stares or admonitions within the context of the group contingency. Furthermore, rewards are naturally occurring or social reinforcers, which cost little and are therefore sustainable across the school year. Although a straightforward and simple classwide intervention, the results of the GBG are striking. A longitudinal research study was conducted wherein classrooms in the Baltimore Public Schools were randomly assigned to receive the GBG, or have business-as-usual behavior management. As expected, classrooms with the GBG had lower rates of disruptive behavior. What was perhaps not expected was that boys from first-grade GBG classrooms had significantly lower rates of aggression in middle school and were less likely to start smoking (Kellam & Anthony, 1998; Kellam, Ling, Merisca, Brown, & Ialongo, 1998). Researchers know that it is often difficult to obtain the effects of an intervention even right at postintervention—to obtain significant effects over 5 years later in a completely different classroom is quite remarkable! It is possible that the GBG promotes appropriate peer interactions and dramatically reduces peer reinforcement for inappropriate behavior early in the child's school career. Structured peer interactions and appropriate behavior management reduce the likelihood of peer reinforcement of inappropriate behaviors (Helseth et al., 2015). Perhaps by modulating this peer ecology through the GBG, primary school teachers have the opportunity to meaningfully shift the trajectory of disruptive behavior development in youth at risk.

Peer Mediation

A frequent setting for disruptive behavior is the school playground or recess area. Children are likely to have more frequent, varied, and complex interactions outside the classroom setting. Furthermore, these settings are characterized by less vigilant and effective adult supervision (e.g., parent volunteers, a small number of adults supervising multiple classes), and there is clear evidence that adults are often ignorant of the extent, severity, and frequency of disruptive and aggressive behaviors that occur (Craig & Pepler, 1998). To deal with these issues Cunningham and colleagues (1998) devised an intervention approach that leverages the peers on the playground as a resource to increase monitoring, problem solving, and effective resolutions within this less structured and socially more complex setting.

Cunningham and colleagues (1998) established a peer mediation team made up of students from across the school. Importantly, even children with a history of disruptive behaviors could be included on the mediation team, ensuring there was diversity of backgrounds. Mediators received approximately 15 hours of training where they learned how to approach students in conflict, address and identify the issues, and resolve the conflict. Following an all-school assembly where the mediators were introduced and empowered by the school principal, mediators patrolled the school playground and were accessible to students experiencing conflict. Using a multiple-baseline design across settings, the investigators demonstrated that physical aggression decreased by 51–65% across the playgrounds observed. Thus, by increasing monitoring of behavior through the student mediators, providing a procedure for addressing conflict when it arose, and instituting the peer mediation procedures as a school-sanctioned and supported program considerably reduced some of the more serious disruptive behavior on school playgrounds.

Discussion of Prevention Strategies

The label "prevention strategies" was purposely used within this section. Although these interventions may be more intensive than typical approaches within general education settings, they are not so intensive that they are impractical for educators charged with a primary mission of teaching (they can certainly be used within the context of targeted interventions as well, and are, but they are framed here as reasonable first steps within intervention approaches). Educators who are motivated to prevent disruptive behavior in the classroom might start with a classwide approach such as the GBG or a similarly constructed group/classwide contingency, and this should reduce overall levels of disruptive behavior within the classroom. Then, more attention can be dedicated to any children who require more intensive interventions such as a function-based intervention, a DRC, check-in–check-out, or a related approach.

Prevention strategies are likely to require continuous implementation. Indeed, these approaches should be woven into the fabric of the classroom so that children are continually reminded of the rules and expectations within the school setting, and they are also receiving an appropriate rate of rewards and positive consequences for appropriate behavior. These programs can also serve as foundational approaches for the targeted strategies that are described within the following section. It is recommended that children with or at risk for disruptive behaviors have preventive strategies implemented first, as these are less costly and intensive than the targeted strategies. For children who respond well to the preventive approach, the more costly resources can be conserved.

TARGETED STRATEGIES

Some children with disruptive behavior disorders will require targeted strategies that are more intensive than the prevention strategies described in the prior section. Targeted strategies are more intensive because they require additional time, staffing, resources, or efforts. Thus, they are multicomponent interventions that typically include a standard curriculum to guide implementation. Targeted strategies may be implemented continuously over long periods of time, or they may be implemented for a specified time period until the behavior is improved to a level where prevention strategies may be considered. Targeted strategies can be used within both general and special education settings, but it is likely that additional staffing will be needed to effectively use these approaches within a general education setting given the time and attention needed to effectively utilize the approaches. The sections below outline a sample of targeted strategies. Because it is a sample, it is important to note that there are other potential targeted strategies that may be used as well and that this section is not intended to provide an exhaustive overview of targeted interventions.

CLASS and First Step to Success

CLASS is a 30-day program developed to reduce disruptive and inappropriate behavior exhibited by children within classroom settings (Hops & Walker, 1988). It encourages the targeted child to exhibit good behavior through a consultant and teacher program. The consultant is the primary implementer for the first 5 program days, with the program gradually turned over to the teacher to implement once the child's behavior has improved. The program begins by having the consultant meet with the parent(s), teacher, and child to explain the program and ensure everyone is motivated to give it a try. Then, targeted behaviors are established for the child and well defined. Rewards for meeting goals related to the targeted behaviors are also established both at school and at home. The consultant then enters the classroom with a card that is green on one side and red on the other side. When the child is exhibiting appropriate and rule-following behavior, the card stays on the green side. However, if a targeted behavior is exhibited that breaks a rule, the card it turned toward the red side. It remains on the red side until the child is again exhibiting appropriate behavior. The consultant begins timing on a stopwatch at the beginning of class and at each predetermined interval makes a mark on the card—on the green side if appropriate behavior is exhibited at that time, and on the red side if inappropriate behavior is exhibited. At the end of the period, the total number of marks on the green side are summed and divided by the total number of marks; if the child meets the goal for green-side marks, the reward is earned.

CLASS incorporates response cost, token economy, control of adult attention directed to appropriate and inappropriate behavior, and group and individual rewards. Furthermore, although there are 30 days within the program, there are recycling procedures wherein a child returns to a prior day's behavioral expectations and has to meet it again before moving to more conservative behavioral goals. In this way the child demonstrates clear behavioral improvements before the expectations and feedback frequency is reduced. Furthermore, the responsibility for program implementation is not transferred to the teacher until the child has displayed 5 days of appropriate behavior with the consultant running the program. When the child is transferred, the teacher inherits a child exhibiting better behavior and a program that requires less intensive monitoring. Prior to the teacher taking over the program entirely, there is also a "hand-off" period wherein the consultant and the teacher partner together to ensure the teacher is comfortable with the procedures and implementing them correctly.

The First Step to Success is a contemporary and expanded version of CLASS that includes an elementary and preschool version (*www.firststeptosuccess.org*). It begins with a systematic screening to identify children who may benefit from the First Step to Success program (see Chapter 2). It includes the CLASS program components as well as a parenting program called homeBase. In this program, parents learn how to support skill development at home through meeting with the consultant or coach. The First Step to Success program has been evaluated and has shown promise as an effective intervention both in the preschool and early elementary school settings (Walker et al., 2014).

Coping Power Program

The Coping Power Program is a cognitive-behavioral intervention that includes child-focused group counseling sessions and behavioral parent training. The program results in significant and meaningful positive outcomes at posttreatment (Lochman & Wells, 2002) and follow-up (Lochman & Wells, 2003). The Coping Power Program spans 2 school years, lasting 16 months. There are 22 group sessions overall, and these group sessions include cognitive-behavioral treatment for youth with aggressive and/or disruptive behaviors. Sessions include teaching the children structured problem-solving strategies, identifying and modulating emotions including anger, social problem solving, dealing effectively with peer pressure, improvement in peer interactions, and study and organizational skills. In parallel, parents attend 16 parent training sessions over the same time period (similar to the approaches described in Chapter 4). Parents also learn the same problem-solving model that the children learn within the child-focused sessions.

The Coping Power Program is intense: it spans 2 full school years and includes a considerable number of parent and child sessions. However, the targets of the intervention include serious outcomes such as aggression, substance abuse, and oppositional/conduct problems. Because these issues are so serious, it is not surprising that the intervention is an intensive one as well.

The Incredible Years

The Incredible Years teacher training program is part of a suite of interventions developed by Carolyn Webster-Stratton (*http://incredibleyears.com*). The teacher training program, evaluated in preschool and early elementary settings, includes components to improve classroom management strategies, improve the social–emotional behavior of students within treated classrooms, and it also includes components to enhance parental engagement with the child in a way to enable academic progress and success. The teacher training program can be used alone or in combination with the child training and parent training programs that are also available.

Multiple clinical trials have validated The Incredible Years teacher training program (e.g., Hutchings, Martin-Forbes, Daley, & Williams, 2013; Webster-Stratton, Reid, & Stoolmiller, 2008). For instance, Webster-Stratton and colleagues (2008) randomly assigned schools to receive the teacher and child training programs or business as usual. Children from schools who received The Incredible Years program exhibited more social competence and fewer conduct problems than children in comparison schools on observational measures where the observer was blind to group assignment. Furthermore, teachers from schools that used The Incredible Years used more positive classroom behavior management strategies relative to those in comparison schools, and they also reported that parents were more involved with their child's schooling. The addition of the teacher training component also appears to enhance and improve outcomes when combined with parent and/or child training components (Webster-Stratton et al., 2004). These results support the efficacy of

The Incredible Years program as an effective intervention for the treatment of disruptive or aggressive behaviors.

Discussion of Targeted Interventions

As mentioned, there are many other targeted strategy programs available for children requiring the most intensive interventions. Each of the programs described above have training, manuals, and support for implementation. Interested professionals are directed to the individual programs for more information. Many professionals may also aim to develop packages of intervention for children with disruptive behavior disorders. This is what has been done within the context of large clinical trials that addressed severe disruptive behavior (Conduct Problems Prevention Research Group, 1998; MTA Cooperative Group, 1999). In both these studies, intensive parent management training (see Chapter 4), school interventions that included partnerships with the teacher to promote effective classroom management (this chapter), and skills training for the youth (see Chapter 6) were combined and implemented simultaneously in an effort to yield positive outcomes.

It should be noted that all of the targeted interventions described are expected to occur within the context of foundational and prevention strategies. Furthermore, it is expected that targeted interventions will be implemented for a sustained period of time and in a consistent manner. Moreover, nearly all targeted interventions will include paraprofessional, related service, or other experts to assist with training, implementation, and evaluation of outcomes. Thus, a team approach is truly necessary to realize gains on this level of intervention.

SUMMARY

On a practical scale, educators can work to implement a multimodal intervention approach within their classroom. Form 5.5 at the end of this chapter is a self-study checklist that can be used to determine which strategies are being implemented currently, which are being implemented but may need some troubleshooting, and which strategies may be worth trying because they are not currently implemented. After completing the self-study, or having it completed after a consultation meeting with a coach or mentor, an educator can begin to change practice in a way that will improve his or her professional approach to supporting youth, especially those with or at risk for disruptive behavior disorder problems.

Daily Report Card (DRC) for Elementary School

Target	Social Studies	English/ Language Arts	Math	Science
1. Completes assignment with time given at 80% accuracy or better.	☺ ☹	☺ ☹	☺ ☹	☺ ☹
2. Has no more than three interruptions during the lesson.	☺ ☹	☺ ☹	☺ ☹	☺ ☹
3. No reports of bullying or teasing from peers.	**YES NO**			
4. Homework folder returned and signed by parent.	**YES NO**			

Parent Signature: _____

Daily Report Card (DRC) for Middle or High School

1. Has no office referrals.		YES	NO
2. Returns completed homework.	Language arts	YES	NO
	Geography	YES	NO
	Spanish	YES	NO
	Chemistry	YES	NO
	Math	YES	NO
3. No instances of verbally abusive behavior.	Language arts	YES	NO
	Geography	YES	NO
	Spanish	YES	NO
	Chemistry	YES	NO
	Math	YES	NO

Parent Signature: _____

Template for a Behavioral Contract

Date: _____

Individuals Present: _____

_____

Issue: _____

_____

_____

_____

Operational Definition of Target Behavior (i.e., behavior to increase or decrease): _____

_____

_____

_____

Behavioral Goal (Specify): _____

_____

_____

Positive Consequence for Meeting Goal: _____

_____

_____

Negative Consequence for Missing Goal: _____

_____

_____

Responsibilities for Plan: _____

_____

_____

Reevaluation Date: _____

_____   _____   _____
Teen Signature   Educator Signature   Parent Signature

Template for a Group Contingency Program

Date: _____

Describe the current problem: _____

_____

_____

_____

_____

_____

Describe how this is a *group* rather than an *individual* problem: _____

_____

_____

_____

_____

_____

Operational Definition of Target Behavior (i.e., behavior to increase or decrease): _____

_____

_____

_____

_____

Behavioral Goal (Specify): _____

_____

_____

Positive Consequence for Meeting Group Goal: _____

_____

_____

Negative Consequence for Missing Group Goal: _____

_____

_____

Reevaluation Date: _____

Self-Study or Consultant Checklist
to Review Current and Potential School Intervention Approaches

FOUNDATIONAL STRATEGIES

Procedure	Use Effectively	Use Ineffectively	Consider Trying
1. Rules			
2. Praise, compliments, celebrations			
3. School-based rewards			
4. Opportunities to respond			
5. Planning ahead for activities			
6. Effective commands and requests			
7. Corrective feedback			

PREVENTION STRATEGIES

Procedure	Use Effectively	Use Ineffectively	Consider Trying
1. Daily report card			
2. Behavioral contract			
3. Function-based behavioral interventions			
4. Group contingencies			
5. Peer mediation			

TARGETED STRATEGIES

Procedure	Use Effectively	Use Ineffectively	Consider Trying
1. Describe:			

CHAPTER 6

Training Interventions in Adaptive Skills

This book focuses on reducing problematic and disruptive behaviors. However, good interventions will always include strategies for teaching adaptive skills. The parenting strategies (Chapter 4) and teacher strategies (Chapter 5) include approaches for improving skills used by adults to manage disruptive behaviors. This chapter targets strategies and approaches that can be used to promote the prosocial, academic, and executive functioning/self-control skills that are impaired within youth with disruptive behavior disorders.

The need for this emphasis on building competencies really hit home for me after working on the case of a child with severe aggression and conduct problems. After working intensively with his parents and teacher, we instituted a DRC, employed a strong reward system at home, and enrolled the parents in a 2-month parenting class to work on their home-based strategies. This work paid off. Soon the child was following more rules at home, the parents were feeling more confident and successful with their parenting, and the teacher reported that the child was handing in homework for the first time all year. About a month after I finished up with the case, the child's father called and said he was really excited by something that had happened that day. His son came home from school beaming because he overheard on the bus that a large group of kids from his class had been regularly getting together to play soccer at the neighborhood playground and he had just been invited. His father was happy about this situation because he knew how much effort had been put in to help the child behave better and now he was being actively included by his peers. This example illustrates how focusing on building skills for the child is just as important as reducing problem behaviors; after all, a child who is happy, socially skilled, and academically progressing is the result by which most parents and educators would call a treatment effort a success. Simply reducing negative behaviors is often clinically insufficient (one reason why parents will stop or resist using medication treatment is because symptom remission it is not necessarily valued as highly as functional outcomes in major life domains; see Waschbusch et al., 2011).

The focus in this chapter is therefore on improvement in functional outcomes. First, the settings and situations where these functional outcomes will be addressed are reviewed. These include the home and classroom as well as after-school programs, counseling sessions, and structured treatment settings such as summer treatment programs. Second, the functional domains that are targeted within skill-building interventions are reviewed. Functional domains include peer and adult relationships, academic activities and progress, and executive functioning. Third, the content of child-based and adolescent-based skill building is addressed. Specific examples of procedures that can be used to promote skill building are provided to guide the educator who is promoting growth in a specific area.

SETTINGS FOR SKILL BUILDING

A tension exists between instructing the child on a particular skill and providing the child ample opportunity to practice that skill in situations where there is a high probability for successful outcomes following the use of the skill. On the one hand, too much time spent on instruction without time for practice is unlikely to result in major behavioral change. On the other hand, insufficient instruction may lead to unsuccessful application, which also is unlikely to result in major behavioral change, and it may lead to the child becoming discouraged due to a lack of payoff from his or her efforts. Thus, professionals must adequately balance instruction, practice, and performance feedback in a manner that promotes the development of small steps that together lead to significant improvements.

The need to generalize newly learned, adaptive behaviors to untreated settings is also critical. Take social skills in peer settings as an example. A child may learn in a counseling session that it is appropriate to enter an ongoing activity started by other children by walking up to the group, asking permission to join, and then join with the ongoing activity. The problem with this approach is it grossly oversimplifies the complexity inherent in peer interactions. Sitting in an office the social skills training includes a basic three-step process: (1) identify the peer group you want to join; (2) ask for permission to join; and (3) start playing with the group once they give permission. Anyone who has been on a grade-school playground knows that the situation the child is entering is considerably more complex (see a related discussion in Chapter 7 about generalization of treatment effects). Children may be starting and stopping games, peers are moving in and out of groups, historical peer relationships and alliances may be difficult to navigate or know about, and the peers could always refuse to include the child in the ongoing activity even if the social skills exhibited were appropriate. Plus, the plan to ask for permission to join the activity is the approach an adult determines is the best one in this example. It ignores other approaches that may be more successful, such as watching until invited to join, joining the activity in progress without asking, starting a new game near the ongoing one, or some other strategy that may be more effective among children of that peer group and age level. These issues are perhaps one reason for the modest to no effect of social skills training for youth with disruptive behavior disorders (see Evans et al., 2013; Pelham & Fabiano, 2008).

One basic principle emphasized in the sections that follow is that children and teens with disruptive behavior will best learn adaptive skills within everyday contexts, not in an office in a one-on-one counseling situation. The one-on-one counseling may be helpful for obtaining youth buy-in to the training, providing some initial explanation, and also coordinating the intervention approach, but it is unlikely to markedly improve functioning. This is because most youth with disruptive behaviors have had plenty of people tell them what they should be doing—if this approach was going to work with anyone it would be with them! That they are still impaired suggests that treatment efforts need to go beyond talk to include practice and application. Performance feedback, troubleshooting, and reinforcement of appropriate behaviors will all be more effective if integrated into natural settings (homes, classrooms, peer groups), and this is also likely to promote generalization as well (see Chapter 7).

PROSOCIAL SKILL BUILDING

There are two main approaches to building social skills for youth with disruptive behaviors. The first approach includes training the child in prosocial skills such that he or she is equipped with knowledge and skills that can be applied in natural settings. The second approach includes using contingency management strategies to encourage the child to exhibit a greater number of prosocial behaviors and a reduced number of antisocial behaviors. Each approach will be discussed and reviewed in turn.

Examples of interventions that include training in prosocial skills include the Anger Coping Program (Larson & Lochman, 2010), The Incredible Years Dinosaur Curriculum (Webster-Stratton et al., 2008), and the behavioral–family systems approach for reducing parent–adolescent conflict (Robin & Foster, 1989). The Anger Coping Program is an approximately 18-session training program that assists youth with disruptive behavior in grades 3–6 in their management of negative emotions, behaviors, and thoughts. The program is intended to be embedded within a school setting, with specific procedures for generalization included in the manual. The Incredible Years Dinosaur Curriculum uses puppets to teach young children prosocial skills. There is evidence it is effective as a standalone program for young children with conduct problems as well as when it is combined with the parent and teacher versions of The Incredible Years program. Finally, the behavioral–family systems approach of Robin and Foster (1989) teaches youth with disruptive behavior how to handle family conflict. This is done through teaching the parent(s) as well as the teen effective communication strategies including the use of "I statements," active listening, and validating the point of view and feelings of others. Furthermore, teens are taught how to use structured problem solving for use in negotiations with their parent(s). Although it can be at times challenging for teens to understand and apply, they are taught about negative thoughts and cognitive attributional errors, and are instructed to use cognitive restructuring techniques to reduce these thoughts.

Teaching youth with disruptive behavior disorders alternative ways to express their emotions may be helpful, especially for teenagers. When angry, many youth may express themselves in ways that only increase conflict. For instance, statements like "You're so unfair!" or "You never listen to me!" or "You don't understand!" typically put others on the defensive as the "you" in the statement ascribes a characteristic or quality to the person the statement is directed toward. Form 6.1 at the end of this chapter provides a worksheet that can be used to help teens identify emotions and formulate "I statements" to express these emotions in an effective way.

In addition to teaching children and teens to use effective communication strategies such as I statements, it is likely that parents and educators will need to prompt and reinforce the use of this skill, among other social skills. Notably, the social skills training studies within the literature that have illustrated positive effects all include a parent or teacher component as well. Pfiffner and McBurnett (1997) trained children with ADHD about the use of effective social skills, while at the same time teaching parents behavior management strategies as well as strategies to encourage, reinforce, and maintain child skill use within the home and in other settings. This study represents one of the few in the literature that indicated a positive effect of social skills training, perhaps due to the active parent involvement in the intervention. Another research team has promoted the development of appropriate social skills through a parent-focused or classroom-focused intervention that teaches the parents strategies for helping support the child in peer relationships. Parents then deploy these strategies while the child is interacting with other children during short, semistructured playdates (Mikami et al., 2010), or teachers integrate the peer-focused intervention into whole-class activities (Mikami et al., 2013).

Prosocial skill building can also occur within the context of intensive summer treatment programs (STPs) or less intensive settings such as after-school or weekend treatment programs. The STP has been identified as an evidence-based treatment for youth with ADHD to address impairments in peer relationships and interactions (Pelham & Fabiano, 2008). On its face, the STP appears to be a typical summer camp with activities including swimming, arts and crafts, sports, field trips, and an academic classroom setting. But interwoven into all these activities is an applied behavior analytic approach that relies on individuals (i.e., teachers, counselors, parents) to implement behavior modification strategies within the natural camp settings—the very situations where peer-focused behavior can be improved and negative behaviors can be addressed if necessary. Across a period of 8 weeks, children have 320 hours of practice interacting with adults and peers in ecologically valid contexts. The STP is a 6- to 9-week program for children and adolescents ages 5–16 years. Children are placed in age-matched groups of approximately 12–15 children, and counselors implement treatments for each group. Groups stay together throughout the summer, so that children receive intensive experience in functioning as a group, in making friends, and in interacting appropriately with adults in multiple contexts (e.g., recreational, unstructured situations such as transitions to and from activities, classroom). A notable aspect of the treatment delivery in the STP is that all interventions occur in the context of typical child and adolescent activities. It is also important to emphasize that weekly BPT training sessions are also a component of the STP. These sessions facilitate parents' development of adaptive and effective parenting strategies that can then be applied outside the STP setting. Child care is typically provided by STP staff one evening per week to facilitate parent attendance at these treatment sessions (see Pelham, Greiner, & Gnagy, 1998).

Treatment delivery in the STP is also continuous. From the moment the child arrives at the STP each morning until the child departs, best practice behavioral interventions are interwoven into all daily activities. There are even clearly specified rules and procedures for mundane STP activities such as bathroom breaks and arrivals/departures. As described in Chapters 4 and 5, antecedents such as the establishment of clear rules for all activities, the provision of clear commands for expected behaviors, and predetermined rewards and punishments are embedded within program activities and provide a framework for intervention. There are also multiple opportunities for youth to observe modeled social skills during group discussions, as well as to see other youth receive rewards and punishments following clearly labeled targeted behaviors. Thus, the opportunities for modeling appropriate behavior and learning about inappropriate behavior and its consequences from peer models are frequent.

The STP has been widely evaluated, and there is clear empirical support for its effectiveness (Evans et al., 2013; Pelham & Fabiano, 2008; for a review, see Fabiano et al., 2014). Many of the procedures used to promote prosocial skills in the STP could also be adapted to be employed within after-school settings or in other settings such as community centers or sports teams. Furthermore, the STP procedures were also part of a multicomponent, prevention intervention program for youth at risk for delinquency and worsening disruptive behavior (August, Realmuto, Hektner, & Bloomquist, 2001), and its use resulted in an altered developmental trajectory. As an effective program, the STP should be considered as a possible cornerstone for any intervention efforts for youth with disruptive behavior who need treatment for peer and adult relationship impairments. A needed area of future work is to figure out how to increase the dissemination, deployment, and eventual reach of this effective intervention.

ACADEMIC SKILL BUILDING

Although learning challenges are not part of the constellation of disruptive behaviors typically identified in youth, they are certainly associated and often co-occurring. It is difficult at times to determine whether the disruptive behaviors lead to increases in academic underachievement, or whether learning disabilities create more challenges in social and school settings, fostering the development of disruptive behavior. Regardless, many youth treated with disruptive behavior will also need support for academic skill building. A comprehensive review of academic interventions is outside the scope of this book; however, some examples of foundational, preventive, and targeted academic interventions are presented here to provide an overview of the different ways these skills can be built within the context of comprehensive intervention.

Foundational Academic Interventions

Similar to the foundational skills discussed in Chapter 5, foundational skills for academic instruction include engaging and dynamic teaching approaches to a lesson, the use of effective whole-class management techniques to focus attention and effort, and praise for correct applications of course content coupled with corrective feedback when the student performs incorrectly (Reddy et al., 2013). Specific instructional support strategies at the foundational level include the use of major concept summaries (summarizing key points frequently), as well as frequent opportunities for the children to provide academic responses to course content (see related discussion of this strategy in Chapter 5).

An additional foundational strategy that can support youth with disruptive behavior disorders is classwide peer tutoring. In classwide peer tutoring, children are paired within a cooperative reading task. These dyads include a relatively stronger reader and a relatively weaker reader who work together on shared academic activities (Fuchs & Fuchs, 1997). The clear advantage of this approach is that it dramatically increases academic response opportunities within the classroom: all members of the class are working on the academic tasks simultaneously rather than one at a time. Notably, the peer-tutoring approach has improved children's ability to read as well as their social behavior in a general education classroom setting (Simmons, Fuchs, Fuchs, Mathes, & Hodge, 1995). An additional advantage of this approach from the angle of managing disruptive behavior is that all children are simultaneously engaged, reducing the impact of interruptions or academic disengagement that may be precipitated by lengthy whole-class lessons.

Preventive and Targeted Interventions

Multiple strategies are available for improving the academic skills of youth with disruptive behaviors. Prior to initiating skill-building approaches, it is recommended that the educators involved first review the strategies outlined in Chapter 5 to ensure that all foundational approaches are in place prior to initiating the more costly and intensive skill-building strategies. Once the foundational strategies are verified as present, the next step is to ensure that the child or adolescent is equipped with the needed academic skills. Table 6.1 illustrates some potential targets for intervention at the elementary and middle/high school level for youth with disruptive behaviors.

An example of a specific intervention for supporting youth with disruptive behaviors in academic functioning is the Homework, Organization, and Planning Skills (HOPS) program (Langberg, 2011). The HOPS program is a 16-session intervention wherein school mental health professionals teach children/teens how to organize their school materials, record homework appropriately and manage homework completion, and plan ahead and appropriately manage time. For instance, organization of the student's backpack, locker, and form repository (e.g., folder, binder) is operationalized for the child using a standard checklist. The school mental health professional teaches the child how to organize all spaces in a manner consistent with the checklist, and then monitors compliance with the checklist over time. Children earn points if the monitoring indicates compliance with the operation-

TABLE 6.1. Overview of Areas That May be Addressed through Academic Skill Building

Functional area	Elementary school	Middle/high school
Responsibility	• Bringing homework to/from school • Having required materials	• Managing short- and long-term assignments • Having all required materials for each class • Remembering deadlines • Recording homework appropriately
Academic content	• Reading fluency • Mathematical calculation fluency • Comprehension	• Reading comprehension • Note-taking organization
Academic enablers	• Persistence with tasks • Attention to tasks • Reducing carelessness	• Persistence with tasks • Attention to tasks • Reducing carelessness • Time management • Managing procrastination • Using efficient study skills

alized checklist; these points can be exchanged for rewards of the child's choosing. To some degree this intervention is consistent with the DRC intervention described in Chapter 5, except that now the target behaviors (e.g., child is prepared for class) are broken down into component parts (child arrives to class with binder; child arrives to class with all required assignment papers; child's papers are organized in appropriate area of binder in chronological order, etc.) and each component part is evaluated for whether it is consistent with the predetermined checklist. This approach to supporting academic enabling skills development has been shown to effectively improve functioning within school settings (Langerg, Epstein, Becker, Girio-Herrera, & Vaughn, 2012), and it is a promising approach for supporting youth with disruptive behaviors as it can be easily integrated within existing behavior management frameworks and daily schedules.

As another example of a multicomponent intervention for promoting academic skills that fits within the targeted category, the Challenging Horizons Program helps support middle and high school students with note taking, homework management, study skills, and goal setting (Evans, Serpell, Schultz, & Pastor, 2007; Schultz & Evans, 2015; Schultz, Evans, & Serpell, 2009; note that the Challenging Horizons Program also addresses social skills and self-regulation, making it an intervention with multiple foci). The Challenging Horizons Program has been implemented both in after-school programs and integrated throughout the school day via school mental health providers. It has evinced positive outcomes on adolescent academic outcomes. Perhaps most promisingly, compared to participants in a business-as-usual control group, those within the Challenging Horizons Program obtained better overall grade point averages, a highly socially valid outcome from the perspective of parents and teachers.

EXECUTIVE FUNCTIONING AND SELF-CONTROL

The area of executive functioning (planfulness, inhibition of impulses, thinking ahead about consequences, directing attention) has been an area frequently targeted in interventions for youth with disruptive behaviors. However, it has also been an area with few promising results. Take, for example, a recent effort to improve working memory, cognitive control, and executive functioning in youth with ADHD using a computer-assisted training program (there are many versions of these programs, but they generally focus on running the youth through a series of tasks to improve executive functioning). Although claims have been made that these programs improve memory, self-management, and effortful behavioral control, analyses of existing data suggest that the effects are modest, if present at all, and that there are flaws within the studies used to support the work (Chacko et al., 2014; Shipstead, Hicks, & Engle, 2012). Self-management interventions for youth with ADHD and related disruptive behaviors that use cognitive control training have also not realized the results desired (Abikoff, 1991). A common theme within these underwhelming self-control and executive functioning training programs is that they are interventions wherein the child or adolescent is removed from the natural environment and trained outside of it with the expectation that the effects of intervention will generalize into the natural environment (see an expanded discussion of generalization in Chapter 7). At this point, decades of research suggest that this "pull-out" approach to teaching executive functioning and self-management skills simply does not work for youth with disruptive behavior challenges.

In contrast, there is some promising support for integrative executive functioning and self-management interventions. A prominent example of this is the Promoting Alternative Thinking Strategies (PATHS) curriculum (Greenberg et al., 1995; Kam, Greenberg, & Kusche, 2004). PATHS is a comprehensive program integrated within classrooms that includes a curriculum for teaching emotional and social competencies that should reduce aggressive and behavioral problems within the school setting. It is taught within the classroom setting using developmentally appropriate lessons and language. Topics include problem-solving skills, knowledge of emotions, self-management, and peer relationship skills. Teachers then continue to emphasize skills throughout the school day in order to help students generalize the concepts and strategies. The PATHS curriculum can be implemented at the preschool level up to the early middle school grades, making it a useful approach for school systems as a universal intervention to promote the development of executive functioning and self-management skills. Results from the Fast Track study, a universal intervention to help support youth at risk for conduct problems, indicated that the PATHS curriculum was effective in improving the peer relationships and social functioning of children who exhibited disruptive behavior (Conduct Problems Prevention Research Group, 1999). The Coping Power Program (Larson & Lochman, 2010) similarly teaches youth with aggressive and disruptive behaviors effective social cognition, self-control, and self-management strategies and then specifically promotes generalization via support from the classroom teacher and parents. These approaches represent the promising areas for future work in the field that focuses on improving youth self-management skills.

Because the infrastructure of many settings (e.g., school, the counseling office, the clinic) is set up for one-to-one therapy or training, the idea of individual self-management and executive functioning training is attractive because it fits in well with a traditional model of intervention. However, the research is resoundingly consistent in that individual counseling or training approaches, absent generalization procedures and integration of treatment components into natural settings, is ineffective. Strategies such as the PATHS curriculum and the Anger Coping Program likely work because they combine training and counseling with dedicated generalization procedures. Such procedures should be integrated into executive functioning programs by school mental health providers.

SUMMARY

A number of interventions are available to support youth with disruptive behaviors in developing and sustaining friendships and appropriate social skills, academic enabling behaviors, and executive functioning. Effective approaches typically include contingency management strategies to promote skills use, and all incorporate parent and teacher training as well to support generalization of skills to situations within the child's environment. Effective means of deploying these admittedly more intensive interventions with community and school frameworks is an area in need of additional study.

Worksheet for Identifying Emotions and Constructing "I Statements" to Effectively Express the Emotions

1. Use this space to list as many feelings or emotions as you can think of: _____

   _____

   _____

   _____

   _____

   _____

2. Next to each feeling above, list behaviors, thoughts, and physical sensations that happen along with the feeling.

   Think about how different emotions can cause the same behaviors or physical sensations— being scared or getting good news can both result in a racing heart, for example. Note that thoughts are usually different meaning that our thoughts can color the way we think about our behaviors and emotions.

   Use the feelings identified above to label "I statements" below.

   - Top issue with: _____

     How do you feel? _____

     What would be a way to improve the situation? _____

     _____

     How could this be said using an "I statement"? _____

     _____

   - Top issue with: _____

     How do you feel? _____

     What would be a way to improve the situation? _____

     _____

     How could this be said using an "I statement"? _____

     _____

   - Top issue with: _____

     How do you feel? _____

     What would be a way to improve the situation? _____

     _____

     How could this be said using an "I statement"? _____

     _____

CHAPTER 7

Maintenance and Generalization of Intervention Effects

In many interviews and discussions with parents of youth with challenging behaviors, a common theme emerges. That is, these behaviors have been around for a long time. Often when discussing developmental milestones parents will say, "He never walked; he was always running." One parent recounted how her child was so fidgety as an infant he broke her nose while she was breast-feeding. Other parents will recall that their child seemed different when she entered preschool, and she was never interested in sitting down for story time or other group activities. These stories are all similar in that the parent acknowledges that the behavior had an onset very early in development. So by the time an educator, clinician, or other professional begins working with the family, the behaviors have been occurring for some time.

Given the chronicity of the behaviors, clinicians must be mindful of this in work with parents. First, it is likely that the parent has attempted a number of strategies to manage behavior already. Professionals should embrace these efforts, as there are probably some strategies that are working or show promise, and the parent can provide feedback on what these are to provide a launching point for intervention. Second, however, there are other approaches that may need to be removed from the collection of strategies used in working with the child in order to realize improvements. Third, this chronicity means that the behavior has been happening for some time, in many contexts, and from a functional perspective is resulting in some benefit to the child (and possibly also for a parent/teacher or family) if it is a behavior that has been maintained and reinforced. This means that treatment efforts are likely to need to be intensive, sustained, and implemented across settings consistently in order for them to result in meaningful improvements. Fourth, professionals should also be mindful that there have likely been other treatment efforts in the past, and, if these efforts have not worked, the parent may become easily discouraged with a new intervention. It is important to consistently remind the parent that change is slow, significant progress is shown through small steps and minor successes, and that effort toward improvements must be maintained over time. True progress is evaluated by looking back over months or years rather than over days or weeks in many cases.

In the remainder of the chapter, some strategies for improving generalization of treatment effects to other settings and for promoting maintenance of treatment gains are discussed. This is important because disorders like ADHD are now widely conceptualized as chronic (American Academy of Pediatrics, 2011). Disorders such as ODD and CD can be managed within the right intervention framework, but they can also cause problematic, chronic difficulties if not addressed consistently over time. Generalization becomes important because problem behaviors may occur in home, school, neighborhood, and other settings. Because of this generalization issue, interventions must address any setting where impairment is evident. This means that a school-only intervention would be insufficient if there are also impairments within the home setting or when interacting with peers in a scouting troop or on a sports team.

GENERALIZATION

Generalization can be defined as exhibiting behavior learned and effectively applied within one setting in another setting where the intervention did not take place and/or contingencies are different. Professionals working with youth with disruptive behavior disorders should explicitly program for generalization, and they should do so in a way that promotes the building of competencies. I am reminded of these issues as I reminisce about the first day I worked in a group setting for youth with ADHD. As children arrived at the program, they played a quiet game of tossing a ball around to one another. A young boy arrived and he interrupted the game by going up to each child, extending his hand, and saying, "My name is Peter; it is nice to meet you." The behavior was polite and the child's behavior was appropriate, but it was abnormal in the sense that all the other children simply figured out another way to integrate themselves into the ongoing game. Clearly, this child was taught that an appropriate social skill when entering a new group was to shake hands and tell the other person your name, and the behavior generalized from the teaching situation to a peer group, but there was a mismatch between the context the child entered and the behavior the child exhibited. This example highlights the complexity inherent in social situations and clearly indicates that professionals working with youth to promote the display of appropriate social skills need to consider this situation if appropriate behaviors that are taught are to be effectively implemented in the settings that matter most for the child: those that occur within everyday functioning (see also the discussion in Chapter 6 regarding office-based social skills training and its limitations for youth with disruptive behavior disorders).

There is some bad news within the literature on disruptive behavior disorders with respect to the construct of generalization—there is only modest evidence that intervention effects generalize to untreated settings, and multiple studies that indicate effects do not generalize. For instance, Barkley and colleagues (2000) studied the impact of interventions aimed at reducing disruptive behavior in students entering kindergarten. In this study there were three treatment groups: a parent-alone intervention, a classroom-based contingency management program implemented by the teacher, and a combination of the two. All groups were compared to a business-as-usual control group. Before discussing the results, I feel that it is important to highlight one aspect of the study: the authors noted that the majority of parents never attended the parenting program. Thus, the dose of treatment intended for the parents to apply within the home setting was not received and implemented. In contrast, the school intervention occurred as intended because the clinicians had strong cooperation from the school district and the ability to meet with the teachers regularly throughout the study. Thus, this study is interesting in the generalization discussion because one treatment was implemented well in the school setting while the treatment in the home setting was marked by poor adherence. If generalization was to occur, the lack of parent engagement should not matter, and the benefits of the school intervention would spill over into the home setting. Unfortunately, this is not what occurred—the study actually indicated very specific intervention effects. The results were interesting in light of generalization in that the parent group did not improve, the classroom-based intervention improved, and the combined intervention improved, but really only for the school-based measures. This study illustrated that at least for behaviorally at-risk children entering school there were not generalization effects of treatment. The take-home message therefore is that interventions need to be actively implemented within all settings where treatment effects are desired.

A second example of the lack of generalization comes from a recent meta-analysis of ADHD nonpharmacological treatment effects (Sonuga-Barke et al., 2013). A meta-analysis is a study that combines the results of all studies in an area together to generate one overall effect across them all. In this study, the authors were interested in evaluating results collected from "probably blinded measures." Basically, these were measures where the rater did not know the treatment received by the child so that he or she would not be biased in his or her ratings to favor treatment. In medication studies this is easy to do—the study includes placebo pills where the medication is not active. In nonpharmacological studies, probably blinded assessments would include a teacher rating completed when the main intervention was a parent management training program. Alternatively, it could include parent ratings following a classroom-based intervention. In the Sonuga-Barke and colleagues (2013) paper, the effect size for measures collected within the setting where treatment was implemented yielded a significant effect. However, the probably blinded assessments yielded no effect. The authors concluded that there was not enough evidence for these nonpharmacological treatments on probably blinded measures, which are more rigorous ways of assessing outcomes. Given the discussion of the Barkley and colleagues (2000) study above, however, it is likely that these results simply indicate a lack of generalization to untreated settings. Thus, there is again evidence that treatments for disruptive behaviors need to be implemented across domains to yield comprehensive effects.

In spite of these findings that treatments for disruptive behavior often do not generalize, there are a few examples of such effects. McNeil and colleagues (1991) enrolled parents of young children (those of preschool and primary elementary school age) within a parent training program. Following the completion of the program, parents reported improved behavior in the home setting. Youth also were reported to have fewer oppositional and conduct problems in the school setting, even though there was no direct intervention within schools, which suggested the generalization of treatment effects for this targeted behavior. In contrast, there was not clear evidence of generalization effects for ADHD-related behaviors or for socialization-related outcomes. Thus, the findings were mixed across outcomes with respect to generalization of treatment effects. Another study examined generalization of social skills training effects for youth with ADHD in sports settings (O'Callaghan et al., 2003). In this study, youth were taught how to engage in good sportsmanship and attentive behaviors within a group kickball game. There was evidence that the children could effectively generalize the skills taught. Of note, one of the strategies introduced was to "train loosely" (see Stokes & Baer, 1977, for a review) in order to expose children to a variety of examples and conditions within which to exhibit the targeted behaviors.

Some of the following recommendations from Stokes and Baer (1977) are still relevant to present-day efforts to promote generalization of treatment efforts: (1) ensure that naturally occurring contingencies are leveraged to continue to promote the targeted behavior; (2) include a wide variety of exemplars in the training; (3) make sure training occurs loosely; (4) make sure information on the contingencies in effect are purposefully vague; and (5) ensure that the stimuli within the training environment and the environment where generalization is targeted share common features.

These principles that promote generalization are useful to consider in the deployment of effective interventions that will encourage generalization to untreated settings. For an intervention aiming to reduce disruptive behavior, to ensure that naturally occurring contingencies are leveraged, a clinician could work with a teacher to promote the use of praise and compliments following the child's display of a targeted behavior. Educators and parents might also ensure that naturally occurring positive consequences occur following the target behavior. For example, when a child raises his or her hand to contribute to a group discussion, if this is a targeted behavior, the teacher might make a point to call on that child to reinforce the appropriate behavior. For older students, a teacher might permit those who have completed an assignment to talk quietly to peers in the back of the classroom. These naturally occurring, positive consequences are the very ones that occur infrequently (or not at all) for youth with disruptive behavior, and it is important to ensure they are present if generalization of gains is a goal.

Including a wide variety of exemplars in the training includes having the child learn about and practice multiple strategies that can be applied across multiple situations. In the example above, where the child shook hands and introduced himself, he was clearly only taught a single exemplar. In contrast, a child who was taught multiple exemplars might be instructed that he may sit and watch until invited, stand within the circle with other children and wait for a ball to be thrown to him, ask if he can join, or introduce himself to the group. By providing multiple exemplars to the child, he or she has the opportunity to develop a suite of approaches for exhibiting the targeted behavior.

Training loosely is related to the provision of multiple exemplars. It involves interacting with the child using a variety of approaches to ensure that he or she is comfortable exhibiting the targeted behavior in diverse situations. This is the opposite of training in situations where generalization is less important, such as answering a home phone, where the same response can be used every time (e.g., "Hello, this is Mary speaking"). Rather, training loosely ensures that the plan for promoting generalization is built directly into the training procedures. Keeping contingencies vague is also important for promoting generalization. This principle is at work when one checks the coin return of a vending machine for a left-over quarter: the door on the coin return makes it unknown whether the reinforcer (i.e., the coin) is in the slot, promoting the person checking to see whether it is there, even if it is a machine that the individual has never been to in the past. A similar principle could be used in training programs to promote generalization by building in random reinforcer schedules to be used in conjunction with the training. Because the reward is present sometimes, but not always, this may increase motivation to exhibit the target behavior over longer periods of time.

Finally, the last point is perhaps the most important with regard to current practice. It is unlikely that one-on-one social skills training conducted by an adult, with a referred child, will effectively generalize to complex peer group settings. This may be one reason why social skills training has not been identified as an evidence-based treatment for ADHD (Evans et al., 2013; Pelham & Fabiano, 2008). Some interventions do implement the training in a situation that shares common features with the setting where generalization is planned. The summer treatment program described in Chapter 6 is one example. In this treatment setting, all training and interventions are enmeshed within classroom, recreational, and unstructured settings (e.g., transitions to and from activities), which provides ample practice and application within settings much like that where generalization is expected to occur (i.e., the child's home and school settings).

A strategy that can be used to promote and track generalization efforts is a DRC. As described in Chapter 5, the DRC includes targeted behaviors. Traditionally, these are operationally defined behaviors such as "Interrupts three or fewer times"; "Has no instances of aggression"; and "Listens to adult directions the first time given." These behaviors, though well defined, help with training loosely as they do not prescribe the specific instances where the appropriate behavior needs to be exhibited. Furthermore, throughout the day, based on the feedback provided by the teacher regarding meeting or not meeting goals, the child will be exposed to a wide variety of exemplars—both positive and negative—to promote generalization of the positive behaviors across situations. Providing a reward menu at home also encourages random rewards for the behavior being exhibited. A side effect of the reward program, and the child's improved behavior, is likely to also be increased natural rewards such as smiles from adults and peers, invitations to participate in class privileges (e.g., spending free time on the computer or taking a message to the office), and positive internal feelings from being successful in the school setting.

An additional generalization enabler may be self-management. Ultimately the goal of all behavioral interventions for youth with disruptive behavior disorders is the self-management of behavior, but this may be a difficult task. Briesch and Chafouleas (2009) reviewed the literature on youth self-managed interventions and determined that many of these are effective. However, it is important to note that the entirety of the intervention was not self-managed. Indeed, adults continued to provide reinforcers for self-managing as well as for exhibiting targeted behaviors. The self-management aspect of the child's intervention involved the child observing, monitoring, and recording his or her own behavior. Thus, it is not well understood to what extent children with disruptive behaviors can wholly self-manage their behavior without adult oversight of the monitoring of behaviors and the provision of reinforcers. This is not terribly surprising because if the child was able to self-manage behaviors, it is unlikely that he or she would be identified as having disruptive behavior disorders in the first place! It does suggest that educators and professionals must be mindful of the limits of self-managed interventions, and though it is a good goal to have the child self-manage behaviors, this should only be done once it is determined that the child is capable of shouldering this responsibility.

MAINTENANCE

As noted throughout this book, disruptive behavior disorders are typically chronic, long-standing conditions that persist throughout a child's schooling. Studies that have followed up youth from an early age (sometimes from birth) through adolescence routinely show that around 5–10% of the sample have persistent impulsive, disruptive, and delinquent behaviors (Moffitt, 1993). In spite of at times intensive interventions, there also does not appear to be sizable effects of treatment for some youth with disruptive behavior, once the intervention is withdrawn (Molina et al., 2009), which suggests a lack of maintenance of treatment effects. Furthermore, it is important to note that parents and educators working with a child who exhibits disruptive behavior might be quite literally exhausted after putting forth so much effect toward supporting and managing the youth's behavior (Dishion, Nelson, & Bullock, 2004). Although it may be a bit disconcerting to know that treatment gains are not necessarily maintained, this is not much different from other areas where treatment is implemented. For instance, a person who stops exercising and returns to a diet high in sweets and fast food is unlikely to maintain weight loss and other health benefits. As another example, an individual who is highly proficient on a musical instrument may find that he or she is quite rusty if he or she has not practiced for a long time. Thus, maintenance must be specifically planned into the treatment process for youth with disruptive behavior disorders to ensure that it is adequately supported once major treatment efforts are reduced.

There are some tips that may be useful for practitioners who are working with youth with disruptive behaviors. The first is to try to implement interventions that are consistent with those already employed by the parents and teachers working with the child. A case study by Fabiano and Pelham (2003) illustrates this approach. Teachers were utilizing a behavioral intervention wherein the child earned rewards based on meeting behavioral goals within each class. This program was maintained with a few minor modifications, including reducing the latency to earning rewards and clarifying for the child and teacher how the child would specifically meet behavioral targets by better operationalizing the criteria for goal attainment. These small changes promoted the implementation of an effective intervention, one that could be maintained effectively across the school year.

Another tip related to maintenance relates to leveraging naturally occurring reinforcers within the environment. In working with teachers and parents, rewards that have to be bought (e.g., video games), or are not sustainable (e.g., payments for appropriate behavior), or are dependent on others (e.g., playdates with classmates) are discouraged. Rewards that are naturally occurring are emphasized. For instance, a child who gets ready for school in the morning may have a choice of breakfast options, or a child who completes all schoolwork within the time provided may be offered free time. A frequent recommendation for homework completion is that as soon as it is done, the child can engage in all other enjoyable activities, something that is both a naturally occurring reward and one that is likely to be sustainable.

Parents and educators may also find it is easier to maintain interventions over time and maintain the gains of treatment if they are coordinated in their efforts. Too often parents and teachers may be in conflict over the best approach to intervention for the child or teen, and this may also happen between parents, coparents, and other individuals responsible for the child's care (e.g., grandparents). If the adults are not on the same page, or are working at cross-purpose, it is highly unlikely that interventions will be effectively maintained over time and across settings. Thus, the adults who are invested in positive outcomes for the child must collaborate, communicate, and coordinate throughout intervention planning and implementation to ensure that any improvements are a result of a shared effort, and that treatment approaches are agreed upon so that they can be maintained.

Although youth with ADHD do not appear to maintain intervention gains, once an effective intervention is withdrawn (Molina et al., 2009), there is evidence that treatments for ODD and CD may evince maintenance of gains, even after active treatment phases. For instance, there is evidence that a sizable number of youth with oppositional behavior continue to exhibit improved functioning, even 1–2 years after a behavioral parent training program has been completed (Reid et al., 2003). One study illustrated that mothers of preschool-age children who participated in parent–child interaction therapy reported the maintenance of treatment effects up to 6 years later (Hood & Eyberg, 2003). These results are striking and they suggest that one outcome of behavioral parent training programs is to actually change the parenting and parent–child interaction pattern in a way that promotes continued adaptive functioning. Perhaps the coercive process introduced in Chapter 2 is reduced or eliminated, sending the family on a different path than the one they had started on prior to intervention.

SUMMARY

Although they may be distal outcomes of intervention, generalization and maintenance are important considerations within initial treatment planning. Professionals need to think carefully about generalization, and ensure that treatment efforts promote the use of skills taught in diverse settings and with multiple individuals (teachers, parents, siblings, peers). Furthermore, it should also be presumed that effective intervention in one setting will not automatically generalize to other settings, and that dedicated efforts toward generalization will need to be employed by those designing and implementing it. Furthermore, there is some optimism regarding maintenance of treatment efforts for youth with disruptive behaviors, particularly in the area of behavioral parent training. For this reason, parents should be involved in most treatment efforts, as they are ultimately the individuals most likely to "carry the torch" across multiple school years and teachers. The strategies outlined in Chapter 4 are a good start for professionals aiming to support parents' skill development as part of a comprehensive model of intervention. A rule of thumb for promoting generalization and maintenance is that intervention has to last for as long as is needed, include all relevant individuals who are working with the child, and that treatment intensity is likely to need to be maintained over a lengthy period of time (perhaps throughout schooling) if gains are to be realized and stabilized.

CHAPTER 8

Medication Interventions

A comprehensive intervention plan for children with disruptive behavior disorders may include the use of medication. School personnel are in the unfortunate role of being the go-betweens in the middle of the prescribing physicians and children's families in many cases. Yet because of their ability to observe behavior within the structured school setting, they are among the best reporters concerning medication effects and side effects, if present. In this chapter medications commonly used for youth with disruptive behavior disorders are reviewed, the evidence for their efficacy in school settings is presented, and a discussion of the role of school professionals in medication management is discussed.

The recent context of medication use for disruptive behavior has changed dramatically due to a series of prominent events that have shifted the approach used to prescribe medication, attitudes regarding medication as a viable intervention for disruptive behavior, and new preparations and administration strategies. These changes have resulted in improvements for disruptive behavior treatment in some ways, but they have resulted in new challenges in other ways. Before outlining the use of medication for disruptive behavior, a brief overview and historical review will help place the recommendations within this chapter in a contemporary context.

Medication use for disruptive behavior was pioneered by Bradley (1937), when it was observed that stimulants reduced overactive and impulsive behavior in youth. Since that time, stimulant medications have been extensively studied for youth with disruptive behavior, typically identified as ADHD, but also with associated disruptive behavior disorder conditions (e.g., ODD and CD). There is clear evidence that medication can reduce problematic, disruptive behavior, at least temporarily (Connors, 2002), and professional treatment guidelines for pediatricians and child/adolescent psychiatrists emphasize the use of medication for the treatment of disruptive behavior disorders (American Academy of Child and Adolescent Psychiatry, 2007; American Academy of Pediatrics, 2011).

Many recent innovations have removed some of the limitations of treatment with medications. They include the development of reliable, long-acting forms of medications (Pelham et al., 1999, 2001). These long-acting medications reduce the need for school-based dosing, which may be an improvement for the youth asked to take the medication. For example, they remove the need for unfortunate announcements over the school loudspeaker at noon to call a child down to the school nurse's office for a "behavior pill." Furthermore, they reduce the number of doses required during a week, which also reduces opportunities for missed doses. Long-acting medication formulations also extend medication effectiveness into the evening hours, which can help children with after-school activities, homework, and rule following within the home setting. Long-acting formulations are now the most common approach for dosing children with ADHD.

The use of medication is not without controversy, however. Parents have been historically loath to medicate children for their behavioral challenges (Waschbusch et al., 2011). Children with ADHD and related disruptive behaviors are also typically unenthusiastic regarding medication due to side effects and tepid attributions of the medication's effectiveness (Sleator, Ullmann, & Von Newmann, 1982). In addition to clear ambivalence or outright opposition from parents, there has been societal push-back against and concern for a perceived overuse of medication for problematic behaviors in children (Hinshaw & Scheffler, 2014). For instance, the largest increases in stimulant medication use have occurred among children—in particular very young children—in the 1990s and early 2000s (though this increase has recently plateaued; see Zuvekas, Vitiello, & Norquist, 2006). Yet, the use of multiple psychoactive medications (e.g., antidepressants, antipsychotics) is increasing (Fontanella et al., 2014). Recent surveys indicate that the majority of children identified as having ADHD are taking medication during the school day (Fabiano et al., 2013; Visser & Lesesne, 2005). Recent research has suggested that children young for their grade in schools are medicated for "disruptive behavior" at a significantly greater rate than older peers in the same grade (Elder, 2010; Evans, Morrill, & Parente, 2010). This raises the question of whether developmentally normal children are being referred for medication treatment to reduce behavioral variability and allow them to approximate the behavior of relatively older peers. If so, this is a serious slippery slope within the area of pharmacological treatment for childhood disruptive behavior disorders as it is not an appropriate reason to introduce children to psychoactive medications and associated side effects.

There have been other recent changes as well. With the advent of long-acting stimulant medication preparations (since around 1998–1999), there has been a significant shift in the way medication is prescribed to children. Prior to the use of these long-acting medications, children often received immediate-release methylphenidate in the morning and again at midday. For many families, medication effects had waned by after-school hours when the children returned home, and parents were left to manage the child solely by using effective parenting strategies. It was therefore not uncommon during this time to meet parents who evinced considerable suspicion about the efficacy of school-day medication because they had not seen the effects themselves. Once medication effects lasted into the evening hours, and parents observed behavioral differences, this suspicion appeared to wane. Although it may have resulted in better adherence to medication, whether there were other consequences of this change, such as less reliance on effective parenting approaches and increased use of medication during after-school hours and weekends, is an area in need of study. A recent study has suggested that introducing children to medication first dramatically reduces parental uptake of behavioral interventions such as parent training if offered later (Pelham et al., in press).

An additional change in the use of medication has been its overall use. Historically, medication was prescribed for use only during the school day. Doctors encouraged medication "holidays" during the summer months or over weekends, and medication was rarely prescribed for after school. When it was used afterschool, it was conventional to use a reduced dose due to the decreased demands present in homes. Prescribers also attempted to use the lowest possible dose of medication that obtained therapeutic effects. All this has changed. Professional treatment guidelines now recommend optimal dosing wherein the prescribers systematically increase the dose over time until the child experiences untoward side effects. At this point the largest dose used prior to these negative side effects is established as the maximally therapeutic dose. This results in the child being prescribed the highest possible dose. Professional guidelines also advise against taking drug holidays, recommending that the child is medicated all days of the week throughout the year. Furthermore, rather than medicating solely for impairment in functioning (e.g., only for school days, only for specific after-school activities), long-acting preparations result in medication being used every day, at optimal doses. It is not hard to figure out that the current generation of youth prescribed stimulant medications is on substantially greater doses of medication, with larger lifetime amounts of use. The long-term consequences of this change in the approach to medication use for youth are presently not known.

PROFESSIONAL RECOMMENDATIONS REGARDING MEDICATION AND ADHD

Parents and providers of children under consideration for medication treatment for ADHD are therefore left with a mixed bag of messages related to the best intervention for the child. The American Academy of Pediatrics has stated that BPT is a first-line intervention for children under age 6 with ADHD. A recent meta-analysis by Charach and colleagues (2013) also reported large effect sizes (ranging from $d = .062-.068$ in methodologically strong studies) for behavioral parent training outcomes in young children under 6 years of age with ADHD. In contrast, the American Academy of Child and Adolescent Psychiatry (1997, 2007) has published two practice parameters for young children with ADHD. Although the 1997 parameters stated, "Stimulants should be used in this age group only in the more severe cases or when parent training and placement in a highly structured, well-staffed preschool program have been unsuccessful or are not possible" (p. 103S), the 2007 practice parameters provided an opposite recommendation: "It seems established that a pharmacological intervention for ADHD is more effective than a behavioral treatment alone" (p. 903), and the prior recommendation for using medication as a second-line intervention following BPT was removed. A parent visiting the National Institutes of Health website would obtain a general and perhaps tepid recommendation for BPT: "Treatment may include medicine to control symptoms, therapy, or both. Structure at home and at school is important. Parent training may also help" (*www.nlm.nih.gov/medlineplus/attentiondeficithyperactivity-disorder.html*). It is likely that these discrepancies in recommendations across guilds and national organizations serve to increase confusion among providers as well as patients. Unfortunately, patient-centered organizations for parents of children with ADHD (e.g., *www.CHADD.org*) do not provide any concrete information on appropriate interventions and sequences of treatment for young children with ADHD, even though these newly diagnosed children are likely to have parents who are most in need of information and resources.

Unlike the at-times contrary information included within professional guidelines and practice parameters for ADHD (American Academy of Child and Adolescent Psychiatry, 2007; American Academy of Pediatrics, 2011), parental preferences are very reliable. Although providers and professional guidelines emphasize the use, at some point, of stimulant medication for ADHD treatment, the research literature consistently illustrates that parents strongly oppose the use of medication, especially for young children with ADHD (Bussing & Gary, 2001; Waschbusch et al., 2011). For instance, a recent study by Waschbusch and colleagues (2011) surveyed parents of young children with ADHD (average age = 5.8 years) using an experimental approach wherein respondents made choices between different combinations of ADHD treatment. Results indicated that 71% of parents' treatment decisions were guided by a desire to *avoid* using medication as a treatment altogether. Further analyses predicted that parents preferred treatments that included behavioral therapy (such as BPT) over medication alone. This study, utilizing sophisticated, discrete-choice research methodology, resoundingly reported that the majority of parents have a preference for nonmedication treatment. This aligns with a large literature on parental preferences favoring behavioral interventions over medication (e.g., Johnston, Hommersen, & Seipp, 2007; Krain, Kendall, & Power, 2005; McLeod, Fettes, Jensen, Pescosolido, & Martin, 2007; Waschbusch et al., 2011), and it would be expected that these preferences for behavioral interventions would be strongest concerning young, newly diagnosed children with ADHD where multiple treatment approaches have not yet been utilized, and medication can still be viewed as a "last resort" intervention.

In spite of some advantages for the current approach to medication, it is important to note there are limitations as well. When I meet with parents to discuss treatment options, there are typically two goals: (1) reduce problematic behaviors (i.e., "fix the problem") and (2) increase functional capacity and competency in key adaptive behaviors (i.e., "build a strong foundation of skills and strategies"). Given these two goals, to use an analogy of a repairman, a provider armed only with medication has a limited toolbox. It would be like a toolbox filled only with hammers. Sure, there might be different types of hammers—some that could pound away for up to 12 hours, some that were intended only for use during a short time, some that had slightly different molecular structures, etc. However, in the end, all that is available within the toolbox are hammers. This is great if you need to pound a nail, but if you have any other task such as cutting wood, drilling a hole, measuring, or holding something in place, a hammer is less useful because it has a restricted range of function. In contrast, the toolbox of a skilled behavior analyst would have a variety of "tools" for not only supporting the child in "fixing the problem" and "building competency," but also a diverse array of strategies for supporting the child's teacher, parents, peer group, coaches, and others who may also need support and/or remediation. Note that medication is typically a treatment only used for the child, whereas behavioral approaches typically support the child plus others within the child's environment. Thus, in the discussion that follows, it is important to acknowledge that the scope of change we can attribute to medication is narrow, and that for most children with disruptive behaviors, if medication is utilized, it should also be expected that additional intervention components will also be employed.

A second issue to consider is where medication use should occur within the sequence of interventions that may be employed for children with disruptive behaviors. There are three main options: (1) using medication and psychosocial interventions simultaneously, (2) using medication first, or (3) using psychosocial treatments first. Each of these options, and a recommendation, is discussed in turn.

Using medication and psychological treatments concurrently has some precedence within the research literature. For instance, one of the four treatment approaches used in the MTA (MTA Cooperative Group, 1999) was an optimally designed dose of medication combined with an intensive collection of psychosocial treatments (parent training; paraprofessional aide in the classroom; teacher consultation; summer treatment programming). Youth who had a high-intensity behavioral modification intervention coupled with medication performed equally well on primary outcome measures to children with medication alone. Importantly, children in the combined condition were able to obtain similar outcomes to the medication-only condition using a lower overall dose, on average. Interactive effects of medication and behavioral interventions for disruptive behavior do appear to be present. In both recreational and classroom settings, there was evidence that a low dose of stimulant medication combined with a low dose of behavioral intervention (i.e., a DRC) resulted in similar behavioral improvements to high doses of behavioral intervention or stimulant medication implemented alone (Fabiano et al., 2007; Pelham et al., 2014).

A second approach is to use medication first. This is by far the most common approach for youth with disruptive behavior, specifically ADHD, after a diagnosis. This approach has limitations, however, as many parents fail to refill the initial prescription, find the side effects of medication to be too unpleasant, or exhibit poor compliance. An additional limitation is that if medication helps the child stay in his or her seat and stop interrupting class, teacher and parent motivation to implement other interventions (academic, social, behavioral) decreases. A recent study that empirically investigated the sequencing of ADHD treatments—medication first or behavioral treatment first—illustrated that almost all parents access behavioral treatments such as parent management training when they are offered prior to medication, but only a handful of parents access parent training programming when offered after medication is initiated (Pelham et al., in press).

Finally, a third option is to implement behavioral treatment first, followed by medication if necessary. This is the preferred approach for many parents, as medication is often viewed as a "last resort." Furthermore, as noted above, much lower doses of medication may be effective if added onto an existing behavioral treatment program. This reduces side effects, the overall dosage of medication ingested by the child, and it may therefore result in better adherence to medication regimens by both parents and children. Furthermore, recent research indicates that not only is this approach more effective, it is also more cost effective (Page et al., in press).

MEDICATIONS FOR ADHD

Table 8.1 lists a sample of medications approved by the FDA and commonly employed for ADHD. As can be seen from the table, the majority of the medications are stimulants, with some recent nonstimulant medications also obtaining FDA approval for use with individuals with ADHD. Of note, although all the medications in the first section of the table are stimulants, effectiveness, side effects experienced, and the length of therapeutic action are not uniform within the same child. Thus, if one stimulant does not work, a second or third stimulant may be tried to see if there is a better therapeutic effect. Furthermore, some preparations are short acting (e.g., immediate-release methylphenidate lasts approximately 4 hours), moderate acting (e.g., Metadate-CD lasts approximately 8 hours), and long acting (e.g., Concerta and Adderall XR last approximately 12 hours). Thus, there are many differences within the class of stimulant drugs often used to treat ADHD and disruptive behavior. These two major classes of medication (i.e., stimulants and nonstimulants) are reviewed here.

TABLE 8.1. Medications Approved for Treatment of ADHD

Generic	Brand name
Stimulants	
Methylphenidate	Concerta, Daytrana, Metadate CD, Metadate ER, Methylin ER, Ritalin, Ritalin-LA
Dexmethylphenidate HCl	Focalin, Focalin-XR, Metadate CD, Metadate ER
Dextroamphetamine sulfate	Dexedrine, Dexedrine Spansules, Dextrostat, Methylin ER
Lisdexamfetamine dimesylate	Vyvanse
Amphetamine, mixed salts	Adderall, Adderall XR
Methamphetamine	Desoxyn
Nonstimulants	
Pemoline	Cylert
Atomoxetine	Strattera
Intuniv	Guanfacine
Clonidine hydrochloride	Kapvay

Stimulants

Stimulant medications are among the most widely used and studied drugs within pediatric populations. Stimulants were the sixth most prescribed medication for youth 0–17 years of age, and prescriptions for stimulants increased 46% between 2002 and 2010, which was the largest increase for any class of prescriptions (Chai et al., 2012). Multiple studies have independently evaluated the efficacy of stimulant medication. Results indicate that parent and teacher ratings of ADHD symptoms are reduced following the initiation of stimulant medication treatment compared to placebo (Connors, 2002). Although the precise mechanism or mechanisms through which stimulants work to reduce the outward presentation of ADHD symptoms is not understood, it is thought that the medication helps stimulate brain functions that are underactive in individuals with ADHD. Thus, although on the surface it may seem counterintuitive to prescribe a stimulant to a person already described as hyperactive, the stimulant medication "stimulates" brain functioning to better organize and modulate behaviors.

Compared to some other psychoactive medications (e.g., antidepressants), stimulant medications have a relatively rapid onset and offset. Stimulant effects are generally apparent approximately 30 minutes after ingestion, and the length of effectiveness spans from 4 to 12 hours depending on the specific product (see Table 8.1). This necessitates daily dosing of stimulants if an ongoing treatment regimen is required. Alternatively, this also allows flexibility in dosing, should a family and prescriber wish to use the medication only for school days or for a brief period of time (e.g., during a sports activity on Saturday morning).

Like all medications, the stimulants have side effects. Common side effects include a loss of appetite, headaches or stomachaches/nausea, and sleep problems. It is not uncommon for a child who takes a long-acting stimulant in the morning to skip lunch and dinner, and then be ravenously hungry around 8:00 P.M. Children may also have difficulty sleeping if the medication is given later in the morning. More serious side effects can include motor tics such as buccal-lingual movements (this is when a child moves his or her jaw in a circular fashion repeatedly or sticks his or her tongue out when opening the mouth wide), eyeblinking, scrunching up of the nose, or shoulder shrugs. Children may also become more grouchy or irritable when taking the medication.

The two most serious potential side effects of medication include risk of reduced height and/or growth retardation as well as sudden cardiac death. In terms of stunted growth, there has been some controversy regarding that question in the past, with studies yielding conflicting results. There has been recent consensus in the field, however, that sustained treatment with stimulants does in fact stunt growth (1–2 cm/year, 0.4–0.8 inches/year) and there is some evidence and concern that these are possibly permanent losses where children do not "catch up" in growth if medication is discontinued (Poulton, 2012; Swanson et al., 2007). A second concern relates to sudden death due to cardiac arrest in children and adolescents treated with stimulants. There is some question about whether there is increased risk due to stimulant medication, with some studies indicating risk and others suggesting no risk (U.S. Food and Drug Administration, 2011). Given this risk, the FDA has recommended that stimulants and atomoxetine (a selective norepinephrine reuptake inhibitor) not be used in patients with cardiac problems or problems with high blood pressure/heart rate.

Nonstimulants

Recently, some nonstimulant formulations have obtained FDA approval. These include atomoxetine, a medication generally recommended as a second-line intervention, after the stimulant drugs, as there are fewer studies on its safety and efficacy (American Academy of Child and Adolescent Psychiatry, 2007). Furthermore, a specific warning for atomoxetine is that a potential side effect includes increased suicidal ideation in children and teens, so children beginning this medication must be carefully monitored for this problem. Other medications include clonidine and guanfacine, which were traditionally used to control high blood pressure. They are now FDA-approved medications for youth with ADHD, but like atomoxetine, they are viewed as second-line medications used only after stimulant medications have been attempted and have failed to yield positive results (American Academy of Child and Adolescent Psychiatry, 2007).

THE ROLE OF THE SCHOOL PROFESSIONAL IN MEDICATION INITIATION AND MANAGEMENT OF DISRUPTIVE BEHAVIOR DISORDERS

Currently, there is a large disconnect between the prescribers of medication (typically pediatricians and psychiatrists) and the individuals who are best positioned to evaluate medication effects (teachers). In visits with school professionals, one often hears the comment that the child with ADHD is "not medically treated," a euphemism for no prescribed medication. Presumably due to busy schedules, urgent behavioral concerns, and the logistic difficulty of coordinating information collection with teachers and parents, many pediatricians simply prescribe medication and titrate up without careful analysis of its effects. Given the careful thought, angst, and consideration parents give to the decision to use psychoactive medication for a child, we as a field can do much better. Below, some strategies to promote the effective initiation, monitoring, and evaluation of medication use are described. It is important to note one qualification: these strategies are best suited for stimulant medications. Alternative medications that are FDA-approved, such as Strattera or Intuniv, require titration and weaning, so the approach would need to be different. It is the position of professional guidelines (e.g., American Academy of Child and Adolescent Psychiatry, 2007) that non-FDA-approved medications for ADHD should not be utilized, except under appropriate physician care following failed trials of FDA-approved medications or in extenuating circumstances.

The first step in medication initiation within schools involves getting all individuals on the same page, including the parents, educators, physician, and even an adolescent if warranted. This is typically best done by identifying a point-person to coordinate all procedures and keep all individuals up to date throughout the initiation of medication. Procedures for this innovative approach were first outlined by Pelham (1993), who describes how to conduct a "medication assessment" for children with ADHD in schools. The assessment is a period of 3 to 5 weeks where the dose of medication and a placebo pill are randomized to each day. Consistent measures are collected across days, and at the end of the assessment period scores for each condition are averaged and compared to determine if there is an effect of medication, whether there is a dose–response effect of medication, and whether side effects were concentrated within any particular dose.

The Pelham approach to a medication assessment leverages the rapid onset/offset of stimulant medications by randomly assigning medication conditions to days. This has multiple advantages over the traditional approach of beginning with a low dose and titrating up. In a traditional titration where the medication dose is stable over a week or month, effects of medication are confounded with anything else that is going on at the same time. Whether it is that the child has a cough or cold, it is school spirit week, or a substitute teacher is leading the class, these factors can influence student performance in school and their effect can be misattributed to the effect of medication. First, by assigning all medication conditions, plus placebo, within the same week, the impact of these extraneous factors are distributed across all conditions equally, providing a clearer test of the medication effects. Second, the random assignment of medication to days, if done in a blind fashion (e.g., a pharmacist packages the doses in opaque capsules), reduces expectancy effects or the chance for bias in ratings.

So, for example, a medication assessment for a particular child could include a placebo condition, a low-dose medication condition (10 mg of a methylphenidate-based product or 5 mg of an amphetamine-based product per day), and a moderate dose of medication (20 mg of a methylphenidate-based product or 10 mg of an amphetamine-based product per day). Through coordinating with the pharmacist and physician, a prescription for five placebo pills, five low-dose pills, and five medium-dose pills could be written and filled. Then, the doses are randomly assigned across 3 weeks of school. (In practice, one nonrandom component is usually included in the approach to the trial to avoid assigning the highest dose to the first day to prevent adverse side effects.) Figure 8.1 offers a sample medication assessment plan for use in an educational setting.

School professionals can assist with medication initiation by collecting a careful baseline of behavioral information so that any medication effects can be compared to prior functioning. There are multiple viable strategies for this collection of baseline information. As outlined in Chapter 3, a number of assessments are appropriate for progress monitoring that may also be useful within the context of a medication assessment. A DRC is one such tool. The DRC is a daily accounting of behavior in all areas of functioning that need to be addressed. Thus, one way to conceptualize it is that it represents *exactly* the areas medication should improve if it is a useful intervention. The DRC is therefore superior to approaches such as symptom checklists as an outcome measure for a medication assessment because it is an idiographic indictor of the child's functioning across key domains. Furthermore, the percentage of DRC goals met each day correlate very highly with more costly measures such as observations or lengthy rating scales completed by the teacher (Pelham et al., 2005). Thus, it is an effective as well as an efficient way to monitor progress and responses to medication.

Day	Dose
Monday—Day 1	Low
Tuesday—Day 2	Placebo
Wednesday—Day 3	Moderate
Thursday—Day 4	Placebo
Friday—Day 5	Moderate
Monday—Day 6	Low
Tuesday—Day 7	Low
Wednesday—Day 8	Moderate
Thursday—Day 9	Placebo
Friday—Day 10	Moderate
Monday—Day 11	Low
Tuesday—Day 12	Placebo
Wednesday—Day 13	Moderate
Thursday—Day 14	Placebo
Friday—Day 15	Low

FIGURE 8.1. Example medication assessment schedule for use in school settings. In this example, a low dose is 5 mg of immediate-release methylphenidate prescribed twice a day. A moderate dose is 10 mg of immediate-release methylphenidate prescribed twice a day.

An additional consideration when starting medication relates to assessing the presence of side effects. As noted above, a variety of side effects are possible, and judgments about behavioral improvement must occur within the context of the side effects of the medication. For example, if a child had a significant reduction in behavioral problems in the classroom, but this decrease coincided with a blunted affect that made the child less likely to participate in or find enjoyment in class activities, many educators and parents would find these side effects to be too costly relative to the benefits related to the behavioral improvement.

In addition to this progress monitoring of medication effects conducted by the teacher, parents should also complete progress monitoring of effects at home. This can include ratings of symptoms and side effects as well as other measures of potential medication effects. For example, parents could use a stopwatch to record the amount of time it takes the child to complete homework each evening. If medication resulted in less time spent on homework, this would be a positive effect of medication treatment. Parents are also best positioned for monitoring appetite suppression or sleep problems, two common side effects. It is also beneficial to include parents in the progress monitoring as this allows the parent and the teacher to evaluate at the end of a medication trial how consistent their observations were for the child's behavior on and off medication. Decisions to proceed with medication, if warranted based on the data collected, will be stronger if all adults are on the same page.

Figure 8.2 provides an example of a school-based medication assessment completed by a school professional in collaboration with a physician, pharmacist, teacher, and parent. In this example a placebo dose, low dose, and moderate dose of stimulant medication were evaluated. The primary outcome measure was the child's percent of DRC goals met each day. As can be seen from the figure, the child met an average of 38% of goals on placebo days compared to 91% of goals when administered the low dose and 88% of goals when administered the moderate dose. Thus, both doses of medication were better than the placebo pill, but not much different from one another. A review of side-effect ratings completed by the teacher indicated that headaches occurred on both placebo and moderate dose days, and that additional side effects were observed when the moderate dose was administered. Notably, no concerning side effects were reported when the child received the low dose, and behavioral improvement was comparable with each of the two active medication doses. After reviewing all the data collected, the team came to the reasonable conclusion that medication did help the child with his behavior, and the lower dose was chosen because it offered comparable behavioral effects to the higher dose, without the negative side effects.

Following an initial medication assessment to determine which, if any, dose is effective within the school setting, periodic follow-up evaluations should be conducted wherein ongoing progress monitoring via the DRC, side-effects ratings, and meaningful outcomes such as grades, discipline referrals (or lack of referrals), and indicators of social functioning are continuously reviewed to ensure that the treatment is comprehensive and maintaining effectiveness.

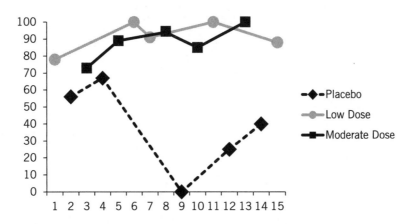

Side effect ratings

Placebo	Low dose	Moderate dose
Days 2 and 9: Headache	None reported	Day 3: Blunted affect; withdrawn Day 13: Stomachache

FIGURE 8.2. Example output from a school-based medication assessment using three doses (placebo, 5 mg dose of methylphenidate, 10 mg dose of methylphenidate).

SUMMARY

Medication is frequently used as a treatment for disruptive behavior in school settings, particularly if a child has ADHD. Medication is often used inconsistently or in a disjointed fashion, however, lacking coordination among parents, pediatricians, and educators. Recent findings suggest that medication is most effective when it occurs following the initiation of behavioral treatments (Pelham et al., in press), and that lower doses of medication are typically effective when combined with behavioral interventions (Fabiano et al., 2007). This is not necessarily consistent with current practice. It is up to educators, parents, and pediatricians to band together to ensure appropriate supports and interventions are in place prior to initiating medication, and if the decision is made to use it, that it occurs within a context of frequent communication and collaboration among all stakeholders within the process.

CHAPTER 9

Targeting Hard-to-Reach Groups

Our current work with youth with disruptive behaviors has focused on utilizing the strategies outlined in Chapters 3, 4, 5, and 6 to address hard-to-reach or previously ignored groups of youth with disruptive behavior disorders. Although the children in the projects all had ADHD, comorbidity rates with other disruptive behavior disorders such as ODD and CD were high. Outlined below are three examples of approaches to support groups that are traditionally underrepresented within the treatment literature for youth with disruptive behavior disorders: (1) fathers of children with disruptive behavior, (2) children within special education placements who exhibit disruptive behavior, and (3) early educators (preschool teachers) who have to manage disruptive behavior on a classwide basis. Examples of treatment materials are included within the chapter; the complete manual for each of these intervention approaches is available by contacting the author.

INCLUSION OF FATHERS IN INTERVENTION PROGRAMS

Parent involvement in school has become a national goal for educators, school districts, and policymakers. The U.S. Department of Education has established an agenda to make schools a central part of the community that incorporate enriching activities for children and parents into the after-school hours, and it has described the "partnership among parents, community volunteers, school staff, philanthropies, and a university" as a key component of the Obama administration's approach to school reform (Senate Hearing, Confirmation of Arne Duncan, January 13, 2009). This is an ambitious and much-needed agenda, but one that requires considerable development to realize meaningful outcomes because educational settings have not typically focused on intervention activities outside of normal school hours.

Chapter 4 reviewed strategies that can promote more effective parenting. Yet, if parents cannot be engaged within the school setting, they will not be routinely attending the school programs that teach these skills. There remains a disconnect between parent involvement in the child's educational experience and parents' (mothers *and* fathers) active collaboration with teachers. For instance, a recent survey of teachers illustrated that whereas 90% of teachers reported that involving parents in school was a priority, 73% reported having an adversarial relationship with parents; furthermore, teachers endorsed the parent as the individual with whom they were most likely to have an unsatisfactory relationship (Metlife, 2005). These results may be even more exacerbated for children with behavioral challenges—approximately one-third of teachers thought parents did not know enough about resources available for their children (Metlife, 2005). Considering general education settings, 65% of mothers are classified as "highly involved" in the child's school, compared to 33% of fathers (Child Trends, 2002); put plainly, half as many fathers are currently highly engaged within their child's school relative to mothers. Results are likely to be even worse within general education settings for youth with behavior challenges due to an ongoing difficult relationship with the school as cited above. It is clear that fathers in general are less engaged with educators in the school setting relative to mothers. Thus, increasing father (this term is inclusive of biological fathers, adoptive fathers, and stepfathers as well as any other adult male in a caretaking role) involvement is a key target within the development of school-based interventions aimed at improving the social and behavioral functioning of students.

One specific area where effective father involvement may result in beneficial outcomes is recreational sports activities. Children engage in recreational and associated social activities in schools during recess, physical education classes, within the classroom, during school-sanctioned sports, and during other unstructured times in school. Organized sports are a context for children to learn important life skills such as working with others on a team, learning to be a good sport, and dealing appropriately with success and disappointment. These sports activities are among the most common things children outside the home experience. It is fair to say that recreational activities are interwoven into the fabric of school settings (e.g., recess, physical education, classroom). Children with disruptive behavior disorders are characterized as having low frustration thresholds, problems with aggression and peer interactions, difficulties with sustaining attention, and following rules, and, due to these behaviors, children in organized sports may present a real challenge to fathers parenting in this setting (e.g., Pelham et al., 1990). Thus, fathers have the potential to contribute positively to child social and behavioral outcomes in these settings (e.g., McWayne, Downer, Campos, & Harris, 2013), yet may struggle without a supportive intervention. Their current involvement in these activities also provides a logical entry point that aims to engage fathers in school-based interventions because it meets fathers where they are rather than attempts to engage them in unfamiliar situations (e.g., parenting classes, in-school meetings to discuss negative child behavior).

Although fathers do not generally play a primary role in many child-rearing activities, they still certainly do have a role. In fact, fathers contribute to many aspects of their child's development, including the development of emotion regulation, social cognition, and focused attention, and—likely because of these factors—appropriate peer relationships (Parke et al., 2002). Fathers who are positively involved with their children have children with fewer mother-reported behavior problems (Amato & Rivera, 1999). Fathers also contribute uniquely to their child's academic achievement and academic sense of competence (Forehand, Long, Brody, & Fauber, 1986). Importantly, these are aspects of functioning that are among the most pronounced areas of impaired development/functioning in children with ADHD.

To simultaneously target the engagement of fathers and promote the teaching and practice of parenting skills, the Coaching Our Acting-Out Children: Heightening Essential Skills (COACHES) program was developed and evaluated (Fabiano et al., 2009, 2012). Specifically, a sports-coaching activity (Pelham et al., 1998) was integrated into the COPE parent training program (Cunningham et al., 1998) in an effort to increase engagement and participation on the part of fathers. COACHES is an 8-week program held for 2 hours each week that integrates sports activities into a parent training program. For the first hour, children practice soccer skills while the fathers meet in a large group and review effective parenting strategies. During the second hour, the fathers coach their children in a soccer game, where they are instructed to practice the parenting strategies they have learned (e.g., praise) within the context of the sport.

The logic model for the intervention (see Figure 9.1) is based on the definition of appropriate father engagement explicated in McWayne and colleagues (2013), which defines two core aspects of positive and effective father involvement: (1) engaging with the child in positive skill-building activities (distinct from basic child-care tasks such as preparing meals, bathing, etc.) and (2) employing quality interactions in the parenting role. The COACHES program directly addresses these two domains through the parent–child interactions in authentic activities (e.g., sports) as well as instruction on best practice parenting strategies. COACHES is hypothesized to be an effective approach because it couples engaging and reinforcing parent–child activities within a sports context with the content introduced in traditional BPT programs. Positive engagement activities include the parent–child interactions during the sports. Quality interactions are those characterized by liberal praise, use of appropriate commands and limit setting, and ensuring interactions are weighted toward more positives (i.e., labeled praise/compliments) and fewer negatives (i.e., reprimands, commands, criticisms). Proximal outcomes of this approach will include improved communication with the teacher/other parent, improvement in parenting skill and increased consistency in parenting, and improvement in the monitoring and management of school performance contingencies. These are all directly targeted within the COACHES intervention. Distal outcomes reflect improvements in child behavior that are hypothesized to result from the improvements in father behavior as well as improvement in coparenting/interparent consistency in discipline related to targeted behaviors. These outcomes include increased academic productivity/homework completion, improvement in behavior/deportment at home and at school, and improvements in social skills and group functioning skills. For coparenting, this is reflected in improved consistency.

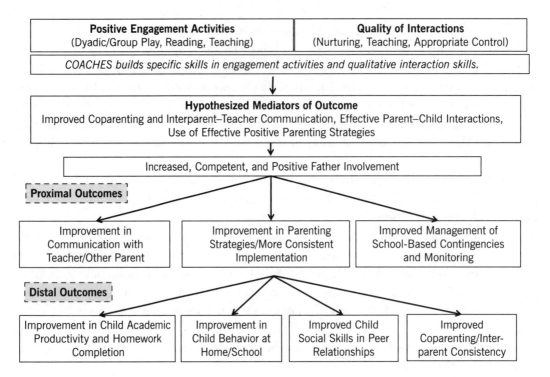

Positive Engagement Activities (Dyadic/Group Play, Reading, Teaching)	Quality of Interactions (Nurturing, Teaching, Appropriate Control)

COACHES builds specific skills in engagement activities and qualitative interaction skills.

↓

Hypothesized Mediators of Outcome
Improved Coparenting and Interparent–Teacher Communication, Effective Parent–Child Interactions, Use of Effective Positive Parenting Strategies

↓

Increased, Competent, and Positive Father Involvement

Proximal Outcomes

Improvement in Communication with Teacher/Other Parent	Improvement in Parenting Strategies/More Consistent Implementation	Improved Management of School-Based Contingencies and Monitoring

Distal Outcomes

Improvement in Child Academic Productivity and Homework Completion	Improvement in Child Behavior at Home/School	Improved Child Social Skills in Peer Relationships	Improved Coparenting/Inter-parent Consistency

FIGURE 9.1. Logic model for the COACHES program for promoting father engagement to encourage school success.

The program has been systematically evaluated (Fabiano et al., 2009, 2012). Fabiano and colleagues (2012) illustrated that the COACHES program resulted in improved outcomes, relative to a wait-list control, by increasing fathers' use of praise and reducing fathers' use of negative talk in laboratory observations. Fathers also rated child behavior problems as less intense at posttreatment in the COACHES group. Fabiano and colleagues (2009) reported results from a comparison of "business-as-usual" BPT and the COACHES program. Results indicated that fathers who participated in the COACHES program attended more sessions, were more likely to complete homework, were less likely to drop out (as were their children), were more satisfied with the treatment process, and at posttreatment rated their children as improved relative to a traditional parent training approach. Form 9.1 at the end of this chapter illustrates an outline of the intervention components during a father–child game session. Form 9.2 is an example of a DRC fathers used to track their child's behavior during the recreational activity *as well as* their own behavior during the activity. In this case, fathers were self-monitoring their use of labeled praise, and their use of this strategy is discussed during each break in the game (see the outline in Form 9.1). Recently, the program has been adapted for use in early childhood settings as a preventive parenting intervention. Parents are provided information on the strategy, its use, and also how to embed it into daily activities including home-based sports practice. The handout in Form 9.3 is an example of the parent materials used in this preventive intervention.

ENHANCING OUTCOMES FOR YOUTH WITH DISRUPTIVE BEHAVIOR IN SPECIAL EDUCATION SETTINGS

The cornerstone of special education services for children with disruptive behavior disorders is the individualized education plan (IEP). The IEP can be conceptualized as an operationalized intervention plan, individualized to meet the particular needs of the student of interest. However, research has shown that procedural faults in the planning and implementation of IEPs exist. Often IEPs are lacking specific, known, evidence-based interventions for reducing disruptive classroom behavior and procedures to increase academic productivity. Thus, many children with disruptive behaviors who receive special education services may be receiving these services inefficiently or the services offered may not be directly linked to important target behaviors that impact a child's learning, achievement, and social development.

In a recent effort, the special education services for children with disruptive behaviors were enhanced by directly linking an evidence-based intervention (a DRC) with the children's IEPs to attempt to bridge the disconnect between special education services and evidence-based interventions. The aim was to enhance the IEPs in a manner that linked classroom behavior and teacher monitoring on a daily basis, to foster daily parent–teacher communication, and to provide a mechanism for monitoring progress toward children achieving their academic and behavioral goals. Figure 9.2 provides examples of how IEP

CHILD 1

IEP Goal/Objective	DRC Goal(s)
• Will continue to improve study skills and work habits.	• Starts work with three or fewer reminders. • Follows directions with three or fewer reminders.
• Will increase basic reading skills. • Will increase basic math skills. • Will increase basic written language skills.	• Completes assignment with 80% accuracy.
• Will develop socially acceptable behaviors.	• Accepts feedback appropriately with no more than two reminders.

CHILD 2

IEP Goal/Objective	DRC Goal(s)
• Will consistently hand in completed assignments on time. • Will self-monitor and self-correct all school work for completion and accuracy prior to handing it in.	• Completes assignment within time at 80% accuracy.
• Will eliminate aggressive/abusive behaviors during all structured and unstructured times of day. • Will use effective coping strategies when faced with conflict situations. • Will decrease outbursts during lessons.	• Keeps hands and feet to self with no reminders. • Has no instances of verbally abusive behaviors directed toward adults.

FIGURE 9.2. Examples of how IEP goals and objectives were modified into DRC targets.

goals and objectives that appeared on the IEPs of two students with disruptive behaviors were modified into DRC targets that the teacher evaluated on a daily basis. Form 9.4 is a DRC that was developed based on a child's IEP goals and objectives. The logic model that was used to develop this intervention is presented in Figure 9.3.

A treatment outcome study was conducted that randomly assigned 63 children with disruptive behavior to business as usual or to an intervention in which a consultant worked with the teacher to turn IEP goals and objectives into a DRC that was sent home each day and with parents who provided contingent rewards for meeting daily goals. The results of this study indicated that the DRC was a feasible, practical, and acceptable intervention. Out of the participants randomized to the treatment group, all DRC group participants completed the study. Analyses to examine the integrity with which the intervention was implemented revealed that, on average, teachers completed 73% of DRCs throughout the entire school year (median = 79%; Vujnovic et al., 2014). This suggests that the DRC intervention can be maintained for a long period of time. Note that all teachers participated, with a median of 79% of DRCs being completed by these teachers, which suggests that for the entire school year teachers completed about four-fifths of potential DRCs on average (Vujnovic et al., 2014). In the study, parents of participants in the intervention group were asked to review and sign the DRC each day and then to return the signed copy to the teacher. Parents returned 64% of the DRC's with a signature (median = 90%; Vujnovic et al., 2013)—note that the median score indicates that nearly all parents returned nearly all DRCs that were sent home with a signature. Parents were also asked to indicate any reward provided, and they indicated a reward for an average of 56% of the returned DRCs that should have earned one (median = 68%). Again, the median suggests that the majority of the DRCs were rewarded.

The DRC condition also resulted in improved child outcomes. Major outcomes from the study included positive effects of the DRC on blind observations of classroom func-

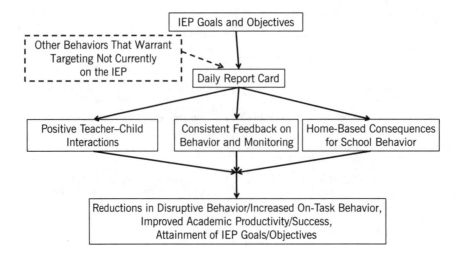

FIGURE 9.3. Logic model for an intervention approach that uses a DRC to help teachers evaluate and reinforce IEP goals and objectives on a daily basis.

tioning, IEP goal attainment, and teacher ratings of academic productivity and disruptive behavior in the classroom. Furthermore, a greater percentage of children with ADHD in the DRC group were normalized on measures of disruptive behavior and impairment—an important finding since one of the goals of special education is to eventually return children to general education if possible. Another important finding of this study was that at the end of the school year, teachers of students in the DRC group were significantly more likely to rate IEP goals and objectives as met, relative to teachers in the business-as-usual group. These ratings corresponded to the blinded observations of student behavior.

The DRC intervention was also deemed as acceptable by participants. Teachers in the DRC condition reported that children were significantly more improved at the end of the intervention. Both parents and teachers noted that the demands of intervention were significantly greater in the DRC relative to the control group, as expected, yet there were no differences between groups on satisfaction with outcomes, supporting the DRC as a viable enhancement to special education services. General and special educators alike could easily take the approach used within this project to potentially improve the outcomes of youth with disruptive behaviors within special education placements.

SUPPORTING EARLY CHILDHOOD EDUCATORS IN EFFECTIVE CLASSROOM BEHAVIOR MANAGEMENT

Teachers consistently indicate that effective classroom behavior management is one of their primary occupational concerns, and it is one of the areas where they feel they are most in need of support and training (Moore Johnson & the Project on the Next Generation of Teachers, 2004). This is especially important when one considers preschool-age children who are new to the classroom setting, particularly those with behavioral challenges. Current approaches to improving teachers' classroom management procedures have been shown to be minimally effective. Many preschool programs utilize strategies such as purchasing books or videos on behavior modification, holding all-school meetings to introduce behavior modification approaches, or inviting speakers for inservices on behavioral approaches. There is currently no evidence that these approaches make an appreciable difference in teacher behavior. The story gets even worse: studies of behavioral consultation in schools, where a professional works with the teacher on a modification of his or her approach to classroom management through consultant–teacher meetings, reveal that the majority of teachers do not even attempt the plan or stop using it in less than a week (Martens & Ardoin, 2002). Therefore, innovative approaches to teaching teachers effective classroom management strategies are needed.

Head Start preschool teachers are required to manage a wide array of situations and child behaviors throughout the day, and virtually every Head Start teacher will confront challenging child behaviors every day. Classroom management procedures can range from implementing a standard classroom routine to responding to serious aggression. In a single morning a teacher may have to deal with students arriving late and hungry, a student who demonstrates fragile toilet-training skills, a student having a tantrum because he did not get his way, the need to coordinate activities across groups with other adults in the classroom, and mediate conflict between other students who are arguing over a prized toy. It is not hard to imagine how difficult classroom management can be within early childhood settings! Because of the need to effectively instruct early educators on effective classroom management, a study was conducted to compare the current approach to teaching early educators how to implement behavior management strategies, a 1-day lecture on the topic, to a more intensive intervention. Specifically, a 1-day summer workshop in effective positive behavioral supports was compared to a condition wherein the 1-day summer workshop was followed by 4 days of an intensive, experiential learning that occurred in classrooms with preschool-age students. All teachers had access to a behavioral consultant during the school year to support their implementation of the strategies within their classroom (see Fabiano et al., 2013, for additional details).

Teachers in the intensive training condition were assigned to teams of three staff (to reflect typical staffing patterns in a Head Start setting). Throughout the day, teams rotated through (1) leading the classroom activities, (2) systematically observing classroom activities led by other teams, (3) providing structured feedback to other teaching teams regarding their use of the effective behavior support skills addressed in the workshop training following their observation, and (4) preparing for the classroom activities. Across the week, teachers had the chance to practice the behavior management strategies across different classroom contexts (e.g., center time, story time, academic tasks) to promote generalization of strategy use.

Each classroom was led by a trainer who supervised the classroom and facilitated feedback sessions. During each of the four experiential learning days, trainers emphasized a particular skill related to positive behavioral supports. These skills, which were presented during the 1-day workshop presentation, were reviewed briefly each morning. The skills emphasized each day were: (1) catching children being good/using positive attention and labeled praise (e.g., "I like the way you are sharing the blocks!"), (2) using effective commands (e.g., "It's clean-up time"; "Please put the puzzles on the shelf"), (3) planned ignoring of minor misbehavior (e.g., not attending to fidgeting at circle time), and (4) "when . . . then . . ." contingencies (e.g., "When you put away these toys, then you can play in the sand table"). Once introduced, a topic was reviewed with the educators each day, and teachers were instructed to use the strategies whenever an opportunity to do so presented itself with the children. In addition to practicing the daily skills, teachers were instructed to use strategies consistent with antecedent control of behavior, and these included remaining on schedule, reviewing the classroom rules before an activity (e.g., "Use an indoor voice," "Walk at all times," "Respect friends and adults"), and also ensure they left enough time for transitions. Teachers were told to provide corrective feedback as they would in their classroom for rule violations that occurred.

When teachers were not leading the activity and were in an observer role, they had a small index card with a checklist of general classroom routines as well as boxes to record teachers' use of the other positive behavior support strategies (similar to what fathers were asked to do during the game in the COACHES program described previously). Once each teaching practice period ended, the teachers who were leading the activities and the teachers who observed the activities met with the training facilitators and reviewed the results of the teaching experience. There, both teachers and observers were guided through a feedback session on the teaching team's use of the techniques. During this brief meeting, facilitators (1) asked each observer to provide a specific example of an instance when the team used the positive behavioral support strategy, (2) asked the teaching team who had been leading the activity to reflect on their opportunities to use behavioral support that they may have missed and to consider what they would like to work on during their next practice session, and (3) provided a summary of the group discussion.

Following the training, observers went into each teacher's classroom in October, February, and May of the next school year. The observers did not know which training group the teacher was in, and they rated the teacher on behavior management strategy use, and they also counted up how many praise statements and commands occurred during the class observation. Results indicated that on observations of effective behavioral management and instructional learning formats, teachers in the intensive condition were improved proximally, with effects waning over time. For measures of teacher use of praise, the intensive group maintained the improved rate throughout the school year relative to the workshop group. Rates of commands and observations of the degree to which teachers used classroom time efficiently (i.e., the degree to which there was downtime for students) were not different between groups. Figure 9.4 provides a graphical representation of the use of praise for each of the two training groups over time. The graph suggests that one impact of the intensive training was to reduce the deterioration of the use of praise over the course of the school

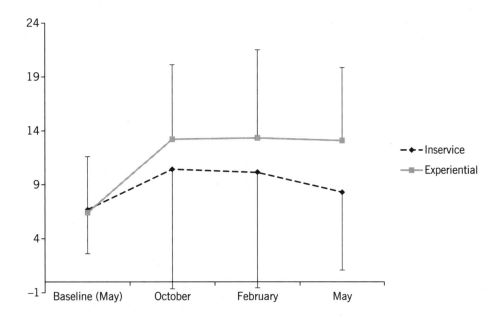

FIGURE 9.4. Graph of teachers' use of praise in the two training groups. One group participated in a single day of inservice training, whereas the other group received the single workshop plus 4 days of intensive, experiential learning opportunities and practice of behavioral management skills (see Fabiano et al., 2013).

year; indeed, teachers in the intensive training started the school year with a high rate of praise and maintained this pace throughout the year. One could speculate that the learning environment of the young children within the classrooms of the teachers who received the intensive training was much more positively focused, and this is perhaps why these teachers also had higher ratings on behavioral management and instruction observations.

SUMMARY

These three approaches to promoting improved outcomes for youth with disruptive behavior disorders provide examples of how the strategies reviewed in Chapters 4, 5, and 6 can be deployed in authentic educational settings. Educators who are confronted by difficult-to-manage behaviors, recalcitrant groups, or other clinical roadblocks are encouraged to view these situations not as barriers to managing disruptive behaviors but rather as opportunities to innovate and extend the reach of effective treatment approaches. It is hoped that the next generation of intervention developments and studies to evaluate them move beyond efficacy trials of school and home interventions to empirical studies of dissemination and implementation approaches to increase the reach, maintenance, and generalization of positive outcomes.

COACHES Game Procedure Sheet
SESSION 2: ATTENDING AND REWARDING

During this session, fathers learn of the reinforcing value of attention, and how praise can be used as a way to make attention rewarding for the child.

Pregame: Program clinicians give feedback to the father on his child's performance on the DRC during the skill drills portion of the program.

Then, assistant COACHES hand the DRC to the father and tell the child that the father is now going to tell the child about the goals for the soccer game.

The father should practice attending to his child. Clinicians tell the father to self-monitor and record all the attention directed toward the child.

Quarter 1: Discuss the types of attention noticed (e.g., praise, coaching, feedback on rule violations, criticism). The assignment for this quarter is to only use praise/coaching for attention. If a child exhibits a behavior that does break a rule, the father must think of a way to praise the child for an incompatible behavior. For example, a child who is not paying attention to the game situation should be ignored. As soon as he or she attends, the father should attend to the child and praise him or her for getting back in the game, etc.

Quarter 2: Discuss with the father how successful he was at implementing the Quarter 1 assignment. For Quarter 2, the father should again practice the Quarter 1 assignment.

Quarter 3: Discuss with the father how successful he was at implementing the Quarter 2 assignment. For Quarter 3, the assignment is to provide positive feedback to negative feedback using a ratio of 2:1 or better.

Quarter 4: Discuss with the father how successful he was at implementing the Quarter 3 assignment. Have the father provide positive feedback to negative feedback using a ratio of 3:1 or better (if the father did not master a positive-to-negative ratio of 2:1 in Quarter 3, repeat the Quarter 3 assignment).

Postgame: Meet briefly with the father and remind him to use his attention and praise contingently during DRC feedback (e.g., attend to and praise goals met enthusiastically and attend to goals unmet neutrally and briefly). Gather the father and the child together, and have them review the DRC.

From *Interventions for Disruptive Behaviors: Reducing Problems and Building Skills* by Gregory A. Fabiano (The Guilford Press, 2016). Permission to photocopy this form is granted to purchasers of this book for personal use or use with individual students (see copyright page for details). Purchasers can download additional copies of this material (see the box at the end of the table of contents).

COACHES Daily Report Card (DRC)

	Skills	Game
Has two or fewer benchings for breaking rules.	Yes No	Yes No
Has no time-outs.	Yes No	Yes No

Children with three out of four yeses earn a cold drink and can participate in a fun activity after the game!!!

Activity Rules (two rule violations in the same category result in a 2-minute benching):	5-minute time-outs for:
Be respectful of others.	Intentional aggression.
Obey adults.	Intentional property destruction.
Stay in the assigned area.	Repeated noncompliance.
Use materials and possessions appropriately.	
Be a good sport.	

	Q1	Q2	Q3	Q4
LABELED Praise				

From *Interventions for Disruptive Behaviors: Reducing Problems and Building Skills* by Gregory A. Fabiano (The Guilford Press, 2016). Permission to photocopy this form is granted to purchasers of this book for personal use or use with individual students (see copyright page for details). Purchasers can download additional copies of this material (see the box at the end of the table of contents).

Parent Handout for a Preventive Parenting Intervention Aimed at Engaging Fathers in Early Childhood Settings

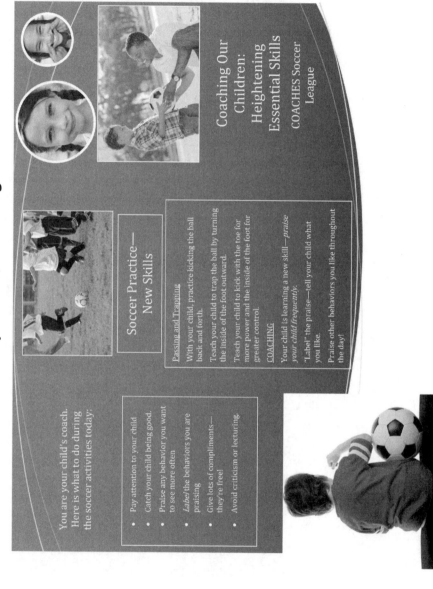

You are your child's coach. Here is what to do during the soccer activities today:

- Pay attention to your child
- Catch your child being good.
- Praise any behavior you want to see more often
- *Label* the behaviors you are praising
- Give lots of compliments—they're free!
- Avoid criticism or lecturing.

Soccer Practice— New Skills

Passing and Trapping

With your child, practice kicking the ball back and forth.

Teach your child to trap the ball by turning the inside of the foot outward.

Teach your child to kick with the toe for more power and the inside of the foot for greater control

COACHING

Your child is learning a new skill—*praise your child frequently.*

"Label" the praise—tell your child what you like.

Praise other behaviors you like throughout the day!

Coaching Our Children: Heightening Essential Skills

COACHES Soccer League

Welcome to the COACHES soccer league!

COACHES is a soccer league to help children and families spend positive time together, build skills, and have fun!

For the next six weeks, your child will learn soccer skills, have fun in soccer-themed games, and you will learn how to coach your child in the sport.

Each week you and your child will each learn a new skill to practice at school and at home. Your child will receive a soccer ball for practicing with you at home.

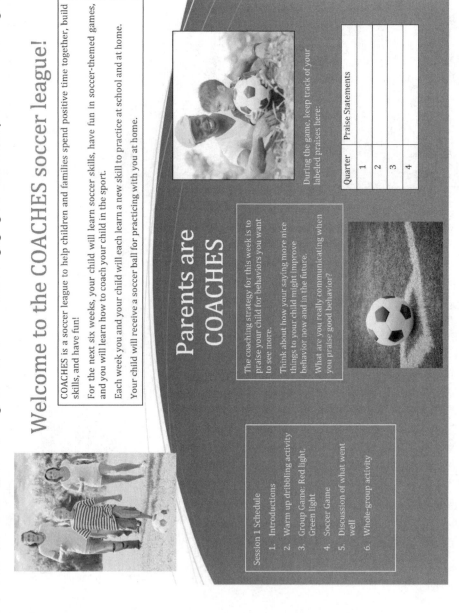

Parents are COACHES

The coaching strategy for this week is to praise your child for behaviors you want to see more.

Think about how your saying more nice things to your child might improve behavior now and in the future.

What are you really communicating when you praise good behavior?

During the game, keep track of your labeled praises here:

Quarter	Praise Statements
1	
2	
3	
4	

Session 1 Schedule

1. Introductions
2. Warm up dribbling activity
3. Group Game: Red light, Green light
4. Soccer Game
5. Discussion of what went well
6. Whole-group activity

Daily Report Card (DRC)
Using Individualized Education Plan (IEP) Goals and Objectives

	Subjects/Times			
	English/ Language Arts	Science	Social Studies	Math
Target 1:	Y N	Y N	Y N	Y N
Target 2:	Y N	Y N	Y N	Y N
Target 3:	Y N	Y N	Y N	Y N
Target 4:	Y N	Y N	Y N	Y N
Other: _____	Y N	Y N	Y N	Y N

Total Number of Yeses _____ Total Number of Nos _____ Percentage of Yeses _____

Comments: _____

_____

_____

_____

_____

_____

_____

_____

_____

_____

_____

_____

_____

_____

CHAPTER 10

Implementing Behavior Management Strategies within a Multi-Tiered Model of Prevention and Intervention

The reader may have noticed that many of the examples from the research literature that are included in this book are decades old (e.g., Barrish et al., 1969; Greene et al., 1981; Patterson, 1975a). This is an important point: the technology and knowledge about how to best address and remediate disruptive behaviors in schools, homes, and communities have been available and well developed for quite some time. This raises the question of why disruptive behaviors continue to plague these settings and cause impaired functioning for the youth and families. One obvious answer is that disruptive behavior typically puts others on their heels, forcing them to rely on consequence control, typically of a punitive variety. As emphasized within this book, school professionals and parents would do well to prioritize antecedent control of behavior to prevent the difficult behaviors from occurring in the first place. One way to do so is through a proactive, schoolwide behavior management plan. These are often conceptualized as tiered behavior management plans such as PBIS (Sugai et al., 1999) or RTI (Fletcher, Lyon, Fuchs, & Barnes, 2007).

One misconception about PBIS or RTI is that it is often presumed that there is only one PBIS or RTI "intervention." In fact, neither is a specific intervention but rather they are frameworks within which interventions are situated, the integrity and fidelity of the intervention is assessed, progress is routinely monitored, and individuals implementing the interventions consciously and strategically modify and maintain the interventions based on the ongoing monitoring system and student progress. Thus, an important realization for school administrators considering schoolwide programming for reducing disruptive behaviors is that they are signing on to a multicomponent, multiyear, and multipersonnel approach to intervention (see, e.g., Owens et al., 2008; Pelham, Massetti, et al., 2005). Indeed, they will need to populate the frameworks with the appropriate interventions within each tier of the framework, and also ensure that the whole organization has signed on to implement the interventions as intended both initially and on an ongoing basis. Anything short of this goal is unlikely to be potent enough to move the needle in a positive direction over a sustained period of time, given the severe impairment experienced by youth with disruptive behavior disorders.

One of the stumbling blocks for effectively implementing multi-tiered frameworks is the difficulty of getting all school personnel on the same page and motivated to implement the new interventions. It is a risk that the new interventions may be viewed as simply another administrative demand, or as a passing fad that will be soon replaced by another set of demands. Atkins and colleagues (2008) recently reported on an innovative approach to disseminating information on treatment for disruptive behavior and also described an effective way to promote uptake and implementation. This project was conducted within the Chicago Public Schools, a large, urban district with many competing demands and directions that may make it difficult to implement new interventions. In the study, all schools had mental health consultants who worked with teachers to help them implement behavior modification strategies that are best practices for supporting youth with ADHD. In some randomly selected schools the consultants partnered with "key opinion leaders" (KOLs). A KOL was a teacher within the school nominated by the other teachers as one of the people they often looked to for advice or as a role model. In the selected schools, the KOL partnered with the consultant to implement effective interventions and also worked to convey the consultant suggestions to teachers. Results showed that teachers in the schools with a KOL were more likely to have teachers who implemented effective behavioral interventions. Furthermore, when additional analyses were conducted, they suggested it was the KOL that made the big difference in implementation, relative to the consultant's contribution (this is consistent with the Martens & Ardoin, 2002, paper that reviews the modest effects of behavioral consultation in schools). This study is innovative in that it illustrates how resources within the schools are potentially underutilized or not utilized at all, and that administrators looking to implement new behavioral strategies might think carefully about how to roll out changes via KOLs rather than traditional methods with known limited effectiveness like faculty meetings or inservice trainings.

So, what else can be done to effectively implement effective behavior management strategies for youth with disruptive behavior disorders? An administrator or school psychologist looking to put together a schoolwide intervention should first survey what practices and strategies are currently being used within the school. A way to complete this survey is to first put together a multidisciplinary team with representation from all school constituents: grade levels, specials classes, facilities and grounds, transportation, administrative staff, and any other group that has an iron in the fire with respect to the effective management of disruptive behavior. Then, the team can work to survey the existing approaches used within the school; many of these approaches can fit within the schoolwide behavior management framework, and others may fit with just a few tweaks (e.g., school–home narrative notes changed into DRCs with home-based rewards). Form 10.1 at the end of this chapter provides an outline that can be used to begin this process.

Using the outline in Form 10.1, an administrator might begin to fill in the tiers with existing interventions. For instance, foundational strategies might include schoolwide behavioral rules; "Good Behavior Bucks" that are handed out to children for following rules in the hallway, cafeteria, and bus line; classwide peer tutoring and other strategies used to manage and direct classroomwide behavior; and a schoolwide demerit system where children receive a detention if they do not hand in three homework assignments. On Tier 2, academic intervention and support groups, "lunch bunch" peer groups to teach appropriate social skills and DRCs might be listed. On Tier 3, paraprofessional aides that float into classrooms may be noted. Following this self-assessment by the schoolwide behavioral support team, the evidence base and effectiveness of all the interventions should be evaluated. For instance, the "lunch bunch" might be removed from the list in favor of training peer mediators to patrol the cafeteria (Chapter 5). A careful analysis might also uncover that although the "Good Behavior Bucks" are frequently handed out, there are no rewards attached to them (perhaps someone on the team recalls that at one point there were actual rewards but things drifted over the years). A principal might also use the opportunity to review the schoolwide rules and add one to address recent difficulties with hallway behavior. In sum, this is an opportunity to take an inventory, conduct a needs analysis, and modify the interventions as needed.

An additional issue that school professionals should be conscious of is the sustainability of the intervention. Too often, one school professional is the champion of a project or program related to behavioral support, and the program lives or dies with this person. We learned a lesson about sustainability when we instituted a cafeteria-wide behavioral intervention to reduce disruptive behavior (Fabiano et al., 2008). The intervention included a reward and response cost ticket system where children in kindergarten through fifth grade earned tickets for random checks of classwide-appropriate behavior and they lost tickets if a student broke a cafeteria rule (e.g., out of seat, yelling). The program was staffed by college undergraduates who earned course credit for implementing and monitoring the system. By all accounts the program was a success because it dramatically reduced the overall disruptive behavior in the cafeteria, which was a big problem for the school prior to the initiation of the intervention. So, given the success of the program, it is not hard to imagine our surprise when we returned to the school for a visit a year later and saw that the current intervention consisted of one of the lunch monitors yelling at the children to sit down through a megaphone! Our intervention was not sustainable because it did not involve internal school supports. From that point on, we have only initiated school interventions that were feasible and palatable to the school personnel currently working in the setting, and we have avoided adding additional personnel that artificially promote appropriate behavior, even if a school requested and was open to this accommodation. This example is a cautionary tale for school administrators to play the long game rather than search for quick fixes because disruptive behavior management is likely to be an ongoing concern that will need continual attention.

There is also more recent attention on implementation and dissemination. A good website on these issues, which includes resources for promoting effective implementation strategies, is *http://sisep.fpg.unc.edu* (see also the discussion of integrity and fidelity in Chapter 3). Once a schoolwide behavioral framework is established, it will require ongoing fidelity and integrity monitoring because within even the best plan there will be drift, accidental "re-invention," or lapses that reduce the overall effectiveness of the plan. Even the most well-intentioned and well-trained implementers are likely to drift over time in their implementation of behavior management strategies, and new situations (e.g., the midyear entry of a student with disruptive classroom behavior who just moved into the district) may require the attention of implementers and supervisors to problem-solve. Ongoing plans for integrity and fidelity monitoring will institutionalize this practice, make it an expected and predictable part of school procedures, and also instill a culture of accountability within the organization, which should help with the maintenance of the program.

Care should also be taken to ensure the developmental appropriateness of the intervention framework based on the school level. Frameworks will have some commonalities across preschool, elementary, middle, and high schools. For instance, some variation of a DRC and/or behavioral contract can be used at each level. Other strategies such as time-out may look quite different based on school level. The frequency of rewards and feedback may need to be more frequent at the younger grade levels relative to the older grade levels. Efforts to engage parents may differ in complexion at the older grades relative to the younger grades. An additional difficulty at the older grades is that middle and high school teachers may view their job primarily as to teach classes to students, given that they might have 120 or more students cycle through their classroom each day. This can be contrasted with elementary teachers who teach the same class of students throughout the school day. This may make more individually tailored behavioral interventions more difficult to employ across teams in the middle and high school, though not impossible. Furthermore, there are strong examples of middle and high school interventions such as the Challenging Horizons program (Evans et al., 2007), which can improve outcomes for these older students.

CASE EXAMPLE

To illustrate the functional approach advocated for within this book, let's return to the child we described in Chapters 2 and 3 who was exhibiting a high rate of problematic behaviors and also experiencing a high rate of negative interactions with parents, peers, teachers, and other school staff. Following a referral of a child like this to the school behavior support team, a problem-solving framework should be used for implementing intervention.

The first step within the problem-solving framework is to conduct an assessment to determine whether adequate foundational strategies are in place and to determine the function of the child's problematic and disruptive behaviors as well as any skills deficits that need remediation. Within this case example, an assessment of the classroom setting is likely to identify increased praise and fewer instances of corrective feedback as needed modifications to the teacher's use of foundational strategies. Rewards and celebrations within the class as a whole may also be emphasized (e.g., through institution of a classwide behavior management approach such as the GBG). From the perspective of the child's functional behavioral assessment, there appear to be some behaviors exhibited to gain attention (e.g., teasing peers) and others intended to avoid tasks that require mental effort (e.g., completing schoolwork). Effective interventions will therefore need to include opportunities for the child to gain attention and also prevent him from avoiding tasks he dislikes through misbehavior.

A DRC is an effective way to organize and initiate intervention in this case. In addition to providing a lynchpin for the intervention approach, it can double as a progress-monitoring tool. Targets are likely to include behaviors that are maintained by attention (e.g., has two or fewer instances of teasing) as well as those maintained by avoidance (e.g., completes math worksheet within the time given; completes all bellwork before the morning announcements begin). Rewards for meeting goals established at home and at school provide an alternative consequence for the child that will result following the meeting of DRC goals. The school psychologist or counselor could also meet with the child's parents to help establish similar interventions at home. For example, if homework time is difficult due to the child's desire to avoid completing assignments each afternoon, parents could be taught to use "When . . . then . . ." strategies to organize homework time (e.g., "When you complete your homework, then you may go outside to play").

Once the DRC, foundational strategies, and parenting support procedures are implemented, should the child still experience difficulties, additional interventions including an after-school or summer treatment program to build skills in academic and peer relationships, or an organizational intervention such as HOPS to promote academic enabling skills. might be introduced. These more intensive interventions would be utilized to help the child build skills needed to continue to make forward progress in school. Although in applied practice additional modifications or supports may be needed, this case example provides an outline of key ingredients that are likely to be needed to realize positive outcomes.

CONCLUSION

This book outlines a set of strategies that can be used to help youth with disruptive behavior. Given the negative outcomes that are possible if disruptive behavior continues unabated, it is critical that all educators, the children's parents, and all other invested professionals (e.g., school psychologists, school administrators, clinicians, pediatricians) band together to ensure each child has an equitable chance to be successful, learn, and ultimately contribute to our society. The good news is there are many interventions that have shown evidence of effectiveness, and, if consistently implemented, should help support the youth who need the help most.

Outline for Organizing a Schoolwide Behavior Management Plan

Tier 1: Foundational	Strategies

Tier 2: Targeted	Strategies

Tier 3: Indicated	Strategies

References

Abikoff, H. B. (1991). Cognitive training in ADHD children: Less to it than meets the eye. *Journal of Learning Disabilities, 24,* 205–209.

Amato, P. R., & Rivera, F. (1999). Paternal involvement and children's behavior problems. *Journal of Marriage and the Family, 61,* 375–384.

American Academy of Child and Adolescent Psychiatry. (1997). Practice parameters for the assessment and treatment of children, adolescents, and adults with attention-deficit/hyperactivity disorder. *Journal of the American Academy of Child and Adolescent Psychiatry, 36*(Suppl.), 85S–121S.

American Academy of Child and Adolescent Psychiatry. (2007). Practice parameters for the assessment and treatment of children and adolescents with attention-deficit/hyperactivity disorder. *Journal of the American Academy of Child and Adolescent Psychiatry, 46,* 894–921.

American Academy of Pediatrics. (2011). ADHD: Clinical practice guideline for the diagnosis, evaluation, and treatment of attention-deficit/hyperactivity disorder in children and adolescents. *Pediatrics, 128,* 1–9.

American Psychiatric Association. (2013). *Diagnostic and statistical manual of mental disorders* (5th ed.). Arlington, VA: Author.

American Psychological Association Working Group on Psychoactive Medications for Children and Adolescents. (2006). *Report of the Working Group on Psychoactive Medications for Children and Adolescents. Psychopharmacological, psychosocial, and combined interventions for childhood disorders: Evidence base, contextual factors, and future directions.* Washington, DC: American Psychological Association.

Anastopoulos, A. D., Shelton, T. L., DuPaul, G. J., & Guevremont, D. C. (1993). Parent training for attention-deficit hyperactivity disorder: Its impact on parent functioning. *Journal of Abnormal Child Psychology, 21,* 581–596.

Angold, A., Costello, E. J., Farmer, E. M. Z., Burns, B. J., & Erkanli, A. (1999). Impaired but undiagnosed. *Journal of the American Academy of Child and Adolescent Psychiatry, 38,* 129–137.

Atkins, M. S., Frazier, S. L., Leathers, S. J., Graczyk, P. A., Talbott, E., Jakobsons, L., et al. (2008). Teacher key opinion leaders and mental health consultation in low-income urban schools. *Journal of Consulting and Clinical Psychology, 76,* 905–908.

Atkins, M. S., Pelham, W. E., & Licht, M. H. (1985). A comparison of objective classroom measures and teacher ratings of attention deficit disorder. *Journal of Abnormal Child Psychology, 13,* 155–167.

August, G. J., Realmuto, G. M., Hektner, J. M., & Bloomquist, M. L. (2001). An integrated components preventive intervention for aggressive elementary school children: The Early Risers program. *Journal of Consulting and Clinical Psychology, 69*, 614–626.

Barkin, S., Scheindlin, B., Ip, E. H., Richardson, I., & Finch, S. (2007). Determinants of parental discipline practices: A national sample from primary care practices. *Clinical Pediatrics, 46*, 64–69.

Barkley, R. A. (2013). *Defiant children: A clinician's manual for assessment and parent training* (3rd ed.). New York: Guilford Press.

Barkley, R. A. (2015). *Attention-deficit hyperactivity disorder: A handbook for diagnosis and treatment* (4th ed.). New York: Guilford Press.

Barkley, R. A., Edwards, G., Laneri, M., Fletcher, K., & Metevia, L. (2001). The efficacy of problem-solving communication training alone, behavior management training alone, and their combination for parent–adolescent conflict in teenagers with ADHD and ODD. *Journal of Consulting and Clinical Psychology, 69*, 926–941.

Barkley, R. A., Guevremont, D. C., Anastopoulous, A. D., & Fletcher, K. E. (1992). A comparison of three family therapy programs for treating family conflicts in adolescents with attention deficit hyperactivity disorder. *Journal of Consulting and Clinical Psychology, 60*, 450–462.

Barkley, R. A., Shelton, T. L., Crosswait, C., Moorehouse, M., Fletcher, K., Barrett, S., et al. (2000). Multi-method psycho-educational intervention for preschool children with disruptive behavior: Preliminary results at post-treatment. *Journal of Child Psychology and Psychiatry and Allied Disciplines, 41*, 319–332.

Barrish, H. H., Saunders, M., & Wolf, M. M. (1969). Good Behavior Game: Effects of individual contingencies for group consequences on disruptive behavior in a classroom. *Journal of Applied Behavior Analysis, 2*, 119–124.

Bor, W., Sanders, M. R., & Markie-Dadds, C. (2002). The effects of the P-Positive Parenting Program on preschool children with co-occurring disruptive behavior and attentional/hyperactive difficulties. *Journal of Abnormal Child Psychology, 30*, 571–587.

Bradley, C. (1937). The behavior of children receiving benzedrine. *American Journal of Psychiatry, 94*, 577–585.

Brestan, E. V., & Eyberg, S. M. (1998). Effective psychosocial treatments of conduct disordered children and adolescents: 29 years, 82 studies, and 5,272 kids. *Journal of Clinical Child Psychology, 27*, 180–189.

Briesch, A. M., & Chafouleas, S. M. (2009). Review and analysis of literature on self-management interventions to promote appropriate classroom behaviors. *School Psychology Quarterly, 24*, 106–118.

Brophy, J. E., & Good, T. (1986) Teacher behavior and student achievement. In M. C. Wittrock (Ed.), *Handbook of research in teaching* (3rd ed., pp. 328–375). New York: Macmillan.

Bussing, R., & Gary, F. A. (2001). Practice guidelines and parental ADHD treatment evaluations: Friends or foes? *Harvard Review of Psychiatry, 9*, 223–233.

Byrd, A. L., Loeber, R., & Pardini, D. A. (2014). Antisocial behavior, psychopathic features, and abnormalities in reward and punishment processing in youth. *Clinical Child and Family Psychology Review, 17*, 125–156.

Chacko, A., Bedard, A. C., Marks, D. J., Feirsen, N., Uderman, J. Z., Chimiklis, A., et al. (2014). A randomized clinical trial of Cogmed Working Memory Training in school-age children with ADHD: A replication in a diverse sample using a control condition. *Journal of Child Psychology and Psychiatry, 55*, 247–255.

Chafouleas, S. M., Kilgus, S. P., Jaffery, R., Riley-Tillman, T. C., Welsh, M. E., & Christ, T. J. (2013). Direct Behavior Rating as a school-based behavior screener for elementary and middle grades. *Journal of School Psychology, 51*, 367–385.

Chai, G., Governale, L., McMahon, A. W., Trinidad, J. P., Staffa, J., & Murphy, D. (2012). Trends in outpatient prescription drug utilization in US children, 2002–2010. *Pediatrics, 130,* 23–31.

Charach, A., Carson, P., Fox, S., Ali, M. U., Beckett, J., & Lim, C. G. (2013). Interventions for preschool children at high risk for ADHD: A comparative effectiveness review. *Pediatrics, 131,* 1–21.

Child Trends. (2002). *Charting parenthood: A statistical portrait of fathers and mothers in America.* Washington, DC: Author.

Chronis, A. M., Gamble, S. A., Roberts, J. E., & Pelham, W. E. (2006). Cognitive-behavioral depression treatment for mothers of children with attention-deficit/hyperactivity disorder. *Behavior Therapy, 37,* 143–158.

Collett, B. R., Ohan, J. L., & Myers, K. M. (2003a). Ten-year review of rating scales: V. Scales assessing attention-deficit/hyperactivity disorder. *Journal of the American Academy of Child and Adolescent Psychiatry, 42,* 1015–1037.

Collett, B. R., Ohan, J. L., & Myers, K. M. (2003b). Ten-year review of rating scales: VI. Scales assessing disruptive behavior disorders. *Journal of the American Academy of Child and Adolescent Psychiatry, 42,* 1143–1170.

Conduct Problems Research Prevention Group. (1999). Initial impact of the Fast Track prevention trial for conduct problems: II. Classroom effects. *Journal of Consulting and Clinical Psychology, 67,* 648–657.

Conners, C. K. (2002). Forty years of methylphenidate treatment in attention-deficit/hyperactivity disorder. *Journal of Attention Disorders, 6*(Suppl. 1), S17–S30.

Corcoran, J., & Dattalo, P. (2006). Parent involvement in treatment for ADHD: A meta-analysis of the published studies. *Research on Social Work Practice, 16,* 561–570.

Craig, W., & Pepler, D. (1997). Observations of bullying and victimization on the playground. *Canadian Journal of School Psychology, 2,* 41–60.

Crone, D. A., Hawken, L. S., & Horner, R. H. (2015). *Building positive behavior support systems in schools: Functional behavioral assessment* (2nd ed.). New York: Guilford Press.

Crone, D. A., & Horner, R. H. (2003). *Building positive behavior support systems in schools: Functional behavioral assessment.* New York: Guilford Press.

Cunningham, C. E., Bremner, R., & Boyle, M. (1995). Large group community-based parenting programs for families of preschoolers at risk for disruptive behaviour disorders: Utilization, cost-effectiveness, and outcome. *Journal of Child Psychology and Psychiatry and Allied Disciplines, 36,* 1141–1159.

Cunningham, C. E., Bremner, R., & Secord, M. (1998). *The community parent education (COPE) program: A school based family systems oriented course for parents of children with disruptive behavior disorders.* Unpublished manual.

Cunningham, C. E., Cunningham, L., Martorelli, V., Tran, A., Young, J., & Zacharias, R. (1998). The effects of primary division, student-mediated conflict resolution programs on playground aggression. *Journal of Child Psychology and Psychiatry, 39,* 653–662.

Dishion, T. J., Nelson, S. E., & Bullock, B. M. (2004). Premature adolescent autonomy: Parent disengagement and deviant peer process in the amplification of problem behavior. *Journal of Adolescence, 27,* 515–530.

Dishion, T. J., Nelson, S. E., & Kavanagh, K. (2003). The Family Check-Up with high-risk young adolescents: Preventing early-onset substance use by parent monitoring. *Behavior Therapy, 34,* 553–572.

Dopfner, M., Breuer, D., Schurmann, S., Metternich, T. W., Rademacher, C., & Lehmkuhl, G. (2004). Effectiveness of an adaptive multimodal treatment in children with attention-deficit hyperactivity disorder—global outcome. *European Child and Adolescent Psychiatry, 13*(Suppl. 1), 117–129.

DuPaul, G. J., & Eckert, T. L. (1997). The effects of school-based interventions for attention deficit/ hyperactivity disorder: A meta-analysis. *School Psychology Review, 26,* 5–27.

DuPaul, G. J., & Stoner, G. (2004). *ADHD in the schools: Assessment and intervention strategies.* New York: Guilford Press.

Eisenstadt, T. E., Eyberg, S. M., McNeil, C. B., Newcomb, K., & Funderburk, B. (1993). Parent–child interaction therapy with behavior problem children: Relative effectiveness of two stages and overall treatment outcome. *Journal of Clinical Child Psychology, 22,* 42–51.

Elder, T. E. (2010). The importance of relative standards in ADHD diagnoses: Evidence based on exact birth dates. *Journal of Health Economics, 29,* 641–656.

Embry, D. D. (2002). The Good Behavior Game: A best practice candidate as a universal behavioral vaccine. *Clinical Child and Family Psychology Review, 5,* 273–297.

Englert, C. S. (1983). Measuring special education teacher effectiveness. *Exceptional Children, 50,* 247–254.

Epstein, M., Atkins, M., Cullinan, D., Kutash, K., & Weaver, R. (2008). *Reducing behavior problems in the elementary school classroom: A practice guide* (NCEE No. 2008-012). Washington, DC: National Center for Education Evaluation and Regional Assistance, Institute of Education Sciences, U.S. Department of Education. Retrieved from *http:// ies.ed.gov/ncee/wwc/publications/ practiceguides.*

Evans, S. W., Owens, J. S., & Bunford, N. (2013). Evidence-based psychosocial treatments for children and adolescents with attention-deficit/hyperactivity disorder. *Journal of Clinical Child and Adolescent Psychology, 43,* 527–551.

Evans, S. W., Brady, C. E., Harrison, N., Kern, L., State, T., & Andrews, C. (2013). Measuring ADHD and ODD symptoms and impairment using high school teachers' ratings. *Journal of Clinical Child and Adolescent Psychology, 42,* 197–207.

Evans, S. W., Schultz, B. K., White, L. C., Brady, C., Sibley, M. H., & Van Eck, K. (2009). A school-based organization intervention for young adolescents with attention-deficit/hyperactivity disorder. *School Mental Health, 1,* 78–88.

Evans, S. W., Serpell, Z. N., Schultz, B. K., & Pastor, D. A. (2007). Cumulative benefits of secondary school-based treatment of students with ADHD. *School Psychology Review, 36,* 256–273.

Evans, W. N., Morrill, M. S., & Parente, S. T. (2010). Measuring inappropriate medical diagnosis and treatment in survey data: The case of ADHD among school-age children. *Journal of Health Economics, 29,* 657–673.

Eyberg, S. M., & Boggs, S. R. (1998). Parent–child interaction therapy: A psychosocial intervention for the treatment of young conduct-disordered children. In J. M. Briesmeister & C. E. Schaefer (Eds.), *Handbook of parent training: Parents as co-therapists for children's behavior problems* (pp. 61–97). New York: Wiley.

Eyberg, S. M., Edwards, D., Boggs, S. R., & Foote, R. (1998). Maintaining the treatment effects of parent training: The role of booster sessions and other maintenance strategies. *Clinical Psychology: Science and Practice, 5,* 544–554.

Eyberg, S. M., & Funderburk, B. (2011). *Parent–Child Interaction Therapy Protocol.* Gainesville, FL: PCIT International.

Eyberg, S. M., Nelson, M. M., & Boggs, S. R. (2008). Evidence-based psychosocial treatments for children and adolescents with disruptive behavior. *Journal of Clinical Child and Adolescent Psychology, 37,* 215–237.

Eyberg, S. M., & Pincus, D. (1999). *Eyberg Child Behavior Inventory/Sutter–Eyberg Student Behavior Inventory—Revised: Professional manual.* Lutz, FL: Psychological Assessment Resources.

Eyberg, S. M., & Robinson, E. A. (1982). Parent–child interaction training: Effects on family functioning. *Journal of Clinical Child Psychology, 11,* 123–129.

Fabiano, G. A., Chacko, A., Pelham, W. E., Robb, J. A., Walker, K. S., Wienke, A. L., et al. (2009).

A comparison of behavioral parent training programs for fathers of children with attention-deficit/hyperactivity disorder. *Behavior Therapy, 40,* 190–204.

Fabiano, G. A., Chafouleas, S. M., Weist, M. D., Sumi, W. C., & Humphrey, N. (2014). Methodology considerations in school mental health research. *School Mental Health, 6,* 68–83.

Fabiano, G. A., Hulme, K., Linke, S. M., Nelson-Tuttle, C., Pariseau, M. E., Gangloff, B., et al. (2011). The Supporting a Teen's Effective Entry to the Roadway (STEER) Program: Feasibility and preliminary support for a psychosocial intervention for teenage drivers with ADHD. *Cognitive and Behavioral Practice, 18,* 267–280.

Fabiano, G. A., & Pelham, W. E. (2003). Improving the effectiveness of classroom interventions for attention deficit hyperactivity disorder: A case study. *Journal of Emotional and Behavioral Disorders, 11,* 122–128.

Fabiano, G. A., Pelham, W. E., Cunningham, C. E., Yu, J., Gangloff, B., Buck, M., et al. (2012). A waitlist-controlled trial of behavioral parent training for fathers of children with attention-deficit/hyperactivity disorder. *Journal of Clinical Child and Adolescent Psychology, 41*(3), 337–345.

Fabiano, G. A., Pelham, W. E., Gnagy, E. M., Burrows-MacLean, L., Coles, E. K., Chacko, A., et al. (2007). The single and combined effects of multiple intensities of behavior modification and multiple intensities of methylphenidate in a classroom setting. *School Psychology Review, 36,* 195–216.

Fabiano, G. A., Pelham, W. E., Karmazin, K., Kreher, J., Panahon, C. J., & Carlson, C. (2008). Using a group contingency to reduce disruptive behavior in an elementary school cafeteria. *Behavior Modification, 32,* 121–132.

Fabiano, G. A., Pelham, W. E., Majumdar, A., Evans, S. W., Manos, M., Caserta, D., et al. (2013). Elementary and middle school teacher perceptions of attention-deficit/hyperactivity disorder incidence. *Child and Youth Care Forum, 42,* 87–99.

Fabiano, G. A., Pelham, W. E., Manos, M., Gnagy, E. M., Chronis, A. M., Onyango, A. N., et al. (2004). An evaluation of three time out procedures for children with attention-deficit/hyperactivity disorder. *Behavior Therapy, 35,* 449–469.

Fabiano, G. A., Pelham, W. E., Waschbusch, D., Gnagy, E. M., Lahey, B. B., Chronis, A. M., et al. (2006). A practical measure of impairment: Psychometric properties of the Impairment Rating Scale in samples of children with attention-deficit/hyperactivity disorder and two school-based samples. *Journal of Clinical Child and Adolescent Psychology, 35,* 369–385.

Fabiano, G. A., & Schatz, N. K. (2014). Driving interventions for youth with attention-deficit/hyperactivity disorder. In R. A. Barkley (Ed.), *Attention-deficit hyperactivity disorder: A handbook for diagnosis and treatment* (4th ed., pp. 705–727). New York: Guilford Press.

Fabiano, G. A., Schatz, N. K., Aloe, A. M., Chacko, A., & Chronis-Tuscano, A. M. (2015). A review of meta-analyses of psychosocial treatment for attention-deficit/hyperactivity disorder: Systematic synthesis and interpretation. *Clinical Child and Family Psychology Review, 18,* 77–97.

Fabiano, G. A., Schatz, N. K., & Pelham, W. E. (2014). Summer treatment programs for youth with attention-deficit/hyperactivity disorder. *Child and Adolescent Psychiatric Clinics of North America, 23,* 757–773.

Fabiano, G. A., Vujnovic, R., Pelham, W. E., Waschbusch, D. A., Massetti, G. M., Yu, J., et al. (2010). Enhancing the effectiveness of special education programming for children with ADHD using a daily report card. *School Psychology Review, 39,* 219–239.

Fabiano, G. A., Vujnovic, R. K., Waschbusch, D. A., Yu, J., Mashtare, T., Pariseau, M. E., et al. (2013). A comparison of experiential versus lecture training for improving behavior support skills in early educators. *Early Childhood Research Quarterly, 28,* 450–460.

Fletcher, J. M., Lyon, G. R., Fuchs, L. S., & Barnes, M. A. (2007). *Learning disabilities: From identification to intervention.* New York: Guilford Press.

Fontanella, C. A., Warner, L. A., Phillips, G. S., Bridge, J. A., & Campo, J. V. (2014). Trends in psychotropic polypharmacy among youths enrolled in Ohio Medicaid, 2002–2008. *Psychiatric Services, 65,* 1332–1340.

Forehand, R., & Long, N. (2002). *Parenting the strong-willed child, revised and updated.* New York: Contemporary Books.

Forehand, R., Long, N., Brody, G. H., & Fauber, R. (1986). Home predictors of young adolescents' school behavior and academic performance. *Child Development, 57,* 1528–1533.

Forehand, R., & Scarboro, M. E. (1975). An analysis of children's oppositional behavior. *Journal of Abnormal Child Psychology, 3,* 27–31.

Forehand, R., Wells, K. C., & Sturgis, E. T. (1978). Predictors of child noncompliant behavior in the home. *Journal of Consulting and Clinical Psychology, 46,* 179.

Forgatch, M. S., & Patterson, G. R. (2005). *Parents and adolescents living together: Family problem solving* (2nd ed.). Champaign, IL: Research Press.

Forgatch, M. S., & Patterson, G. R. (2010). Parent Management Training—Oregon Model: An intervention for antisocial behavior in children and adolescents. In J. R. Weisz & A. E. Kazdin (Eds.), *Evidence-based psychotherapies for children and adolescents* (2nd ed., pp. 159–178). New York: Guilford Press.

Fuchs, D., & Fuchs, L. S. (1997). Peer-assisted learning strategies: Making classrooms more responsive to diversity. *American Education Research Journal, 34,* 174–206.

Goodman, A., & Goodman, R. (2009). Strengths and Difficulties Questionnaire as a dimensional measure of child mental health. *Journal of the American Academy of Child and Adolescent Psychiatry, 48,* 400–403.

Goodman, R. (1997). The Strengths and Difficulties Questionnaire: A research note. *Journal of Child Psychology and Psychiatry, 38,* 581–586.

Goodman, R. (2001). Psychometric properties of the Strengths and Difficulties Questionnaire (SDQ). *Journal of the American Academy of Child and Adolescent Psychiatry, 40,* 1337–1345.

Gottman, J., Notarius, C., Gonso, J., & Markman, H. (1976). *A couple's guide to communication.* Champaign, IL: Research Press.

Greenberg, M. T., Kusché, C. A., Cook, E. T., & Quamma, J. P. (1995). Promoting emotional competence in school-aged children: The effects of the PATHS curriculum. *Development and Psychopathology, 7,* 117–136.

Greene, B. F., Bailey, J. S., & Barber, F. (1981). An analysis and reduction of disruptive behavior on school buses. *Journal of Applied Behavior Analysis, 14,* 177–192.

Gresham, F. M. (2015). *Disruptive behavior disorders: Evidence-based practice for assessment and intervention.* New York: Guilford Press.

Gresham, F. M., Reschly, D. J., & Carey, M. P. (1987). Teachers as "tests": Classification accuracy and concurrent validation in the identification of learning disabled children. *School Psychology Review, 16,* 543–553.

Hanf, C. (1969, April). *A two stage program for modifying maternal controlling during the mother–child interaction.* Paper presented at the annual meeting of the Western Psychological Association, Vancouver, BC, Canada.

Hartman, R. R., Stage, S. A., & Webster-Stratton, C. (2003). A growth curve analysis of parent training outcomes: Examining the influence of child risk factors (inattention, impulsivity, and hyperactivity problems), parental and family risk factors. *Journal of Child Psychology and Psychiatry, 44,* 388–398.

Helseth, S. A., Waschbusch, D. A., Gnagy, E. M., Onyango, A. N., Burrows-MacLean, L., Fabiano, G. A., et al. (2015). Effects of behavioral and pharmacological therapies on peer reinforcement of deviancy in children with ADHD-only, ADHD and conduct problems, and controls. *Journal of Consulting and Clinical Psychology, 83*(2), 280–292.

Hemmeter, M. L., Fox, L., Jack, S., & Broyles, L. (2007). A program-wide model of positive behavior support in early childhood settings. *Journal of Early Interventions, 29,* 337–355.

Hinshaw, S. P., Owens, E. B., Wells, K. C., Kraemer, H. C., Abikoff, H. B., Arnold, L. E., et al. (2000). Family processes and treatment outcome in the MTA: Negative/ineffective parenting practices in relation to multimodal treatment. *Journal of Abnormal Child Psychology, 28,* 555–568.

Hinshaw, S. P., & Scheffler, R. M. (2014). *The ADHD explosion: Myths, medication, money, and today's push for performance.* New York: Oxford University Press.

Hoath, F. E., & Sanders, M. R. (2002). A feasibility study of enhanced group Triple P-Positive Parenting Program for parents of children with attention-deficit/hyperactivity disorder. *Behaviour Change, 19,* 191–206.

Hobbs, S. A., & Forehand, R. (1977). Important parameters in the use of timeout with children: A re-examination. *Journal of Behavior Therapy and Experimental Psychiatry, 8,* 365–370.

Hood, K. K., & Eyberg, S. M. (2003). Outcomes of parent–child interaction therapy: Mothers' reports of maintenance three to six years after treatment. *Journal of Clinical Child and Adolescent Psychology, 32,* 419–429.

Hops, H., & Walker, H. M. (1988). *CLASS: Contingencies for Learning and Academic and Social Skills.* Seattle, WA: Educational Achievement Systems.

Hops, H., Walker, H. M., Hernandez Fleischman, D., Nagoshi, J. T., Omura, R. T., Skindrud, K., et al. (2013). A randomized controlled trial of the impact of a teacher management program on the classroom behavior of children with and without behavior problems. *Journal of School Psychology, 51,* 571–585.

Hutchings, J., Martin-Forbes, P., Daley, D., & Williams, M. E. (2013). A randomized controlled trial of the impact of a teacher classroom management program on the classroom behavior of children with and without behavior problems. *Journal of School Psychology, 51,* 571–585.

Jensen, P. S., Arnold, L. E., Swanson, J. M., Vitiello, B., Abikoff, H. B., Greenhill, L. L., et al. (2007). 3-year follow-up of the NIMH MTA study. *Journal of the American Academy of Child and Adolescent Psychiatry, 46,* 989–1002.

Johnston, C., Hommersen, P., & Seipp, C. (2007). Acceptability of behavioral and pharmacological treatments for attention-deficit/hyperactivity disorder: Relations to child and parent characteristics. *Behavior Therapy, 39,* 22–32.

Johnston, C., & Mah, J. W. T. (2008). Child attention-deficit/hyperactivity disorder. In J. Hunsley & E. J. Mash (Eds.), *A guide to assessments that work* (pp. 17–40). New York: Oxford University Press.

Kam, C. M., Greenberg, M. T., & Kusche, C. A. (2004). Sustained effects of the PATHS curriculum on the social and psychological adjustment of children in special education. *Journal of Emotional and Behavioral Disorders, 12,* 66–78.

Kellam, S. G., & Anthony, J. C. (1998). Targeting early antecedents to prevent tobacco smoking: Findings from an epidemiologically based randomized field trial. *American Journal of Public Health, 88,* 1490–1495.

Kellam, S. G., Ling, X., Merisca, R., Brown, C. H., & Ialongo, N. (1998). The effect of the level of aggression in the first grade classroom on the course and malleability of aggressive behavior into middle school. *Development and Psychopathology, 10,* 165–185.

Kelley, M. L. (1990). *School–home notes: Promoting children's classroom success.* New York: Guilford Press.

Kilgus, S. P., Chafouleas, S. M., & Riley-Tillman, T. C. (2013). Development and initial validation of the Social and Academic Behavior Risk Screener for elementary grades. *School Psychology Quarterly, 28,* 210–226.

Kilgus, S. P., Riley-Tillman, T. C., Chafouleas, S. M., Christ, T. J., & Welsh, M. E. (2014). Direct behavior rating as a school-based behavior universal screener: Replication across sites. *Journal of School Psychology, 52,* 63–82.

Klein, R. G., & Abikoff, H. (1997). Behavior therapy and methylphenidate in the treatment of children with ADHD. *Journal of Attention Disorders, 2,* 89–114.

Krain, A. L., Kendall, P. C., & Power, T. J. (2005). The role of treatment acceptability in the initiation of treatment for ADHD. *Journal of Attention Disorders, 9,* 425–434.

Lane, K. L., Menzies, H. M., Bruhn, A. L., & Crnobori, M. (2010). *Managing challenging behaviors in schools: Research-based strategies that work.* New York: Guilford Press.

Langberg, J. M. (2011). *Homework, organization, and planning skills (HOPS) interventions: A treatment manual.* Bethesda, MD: National Association of School Psychologists.

Langberg, J. M., Epstein, J. N., Becker, S. P., Girio-Herrera, E., & Vaughn, A. J. (2012). Evaluation of the Homework, Organization, and Planning Skills (HOPS) intervention for middle school students with attention deficit hyperactivity disorder as implemented by school mental health providers. *School Psychology Review, 41,* 342–364.

Larson, J., & Lochman, J. E. (2010). *Helping schoolchildren cope with anger: A cognitive behavioral intervention* (2nd ed.). New York: Guilford Press.

Lewinsohn, P. M., Antonuccio, D., Steinmetz, J., & Teri, L. (1984). *The Coping with Depression Course: A psychoeducational intervention for unipolar depression.* Eugene, OR: Castalia.

Lewis, R. (2001). Classroom discipline and student responsibility: The students' view. *Teaching and Teacher Education, 17,* 307–319.

Lochman, J. E., & Wells, K. C. (2002). The Coping Power program at the middle school transition: Universal and indicated prevention effects. *Psychology of Addictive Behaviors, 16,* S40–S54.

Lochman, J. E., & Wells, K. C. (2003). Effectiveness of the Coping Power program and of classroom intervention with aggressive children: Outcomes at a 1-year follow-up. *Behavior Therapy, 34,* 493–515.

Lundahl, B., Risser, H. J., & Lovejoy, M. C. (2006). A meta-analysis of parent training: Moderators and follow-up effects. *Clinical Psychology Review, 26,* 86–104.

MacDonough, T. S., & Forehand, R. (1973). Response-contingent time out: Important parameters in behavior modification with children. *Journal of Behavior Therapy and Experimental Psychiatry, 4,* 231–236.

Madsen, C. H., Becker, W. C., & Thomas, D. R. (1968). Rules, praise, and ignoring: Elements of elementary classroom control. *Journal of Applied Behavior Analysis, 1,* 139–150.

Maggin, D. M., Johnson, A. H., Chafouleas, S. M., Ruberto, L. M., & Berggren, M. (2012). A systematic evidence review of school-based group contingency interventions for students with challenging behavior. *Journal of School Psychology, 50,* 625–654.

Mannuzza, S., & Klein, R. G. (1998). Adolescent and adult outcomes in attention-deficit/hyperactivity disorder. In H. C. Quay & A. E. Hogan (Eds.), *Handbook of disruptive behavior disorders* (pp. 279–294). New York: Kluwer Academic/Plenum Press.

Martens, B. K., & Ardoin, S. P. (2002). Training school psychologists in behavior support consultation. *Child and Family Behavior Therapy, 24,* 147–163.

Mash, E. J., & Hunsley, J. (2008). Evidence-based assessment of child and adolescent disorders: Issues and challenges. *Journal of Clinical Child and Adolescent Psychology, 34,* 362–379.

McCleary, L., & Ridley, T. (1999). Parenting adolescents with ADHD: Evaluation of a psychoeducation group. *Patient Education and Counseling, 38,* 3–10.

McDonald, M. R., & Budd, K. S. (1983). "Booster shots" following didactic parent training: Effects of follow-up using graphic feedback and instructions. *Behavior Modification, 7,* 211–223.

McLeod, J. D., Fettes, D. L., Jensen, P. S., Pescosolido, B. A., & Martin, J. K. (2007). Public knowledge, beliefs, and treatment preferences concerning attention-deficit/hyperactivity disorder. *Psychiatric Services, 58,* 626–631.

McMahon, R. J., & Forehand, R. (2005). *Helping the noncompliant child: Family-based treatment for oppositional behavior.* New York: Guilford Press.

McMahon, R. J., & Frick, P. J. (2005). Evidence-based assessment of conduct problems in children and adolescents. *Journal of Clinical Child and Adolescent Psychology, 34,* 477–505.

McNeil, C. B., Eyberg, S., Eisenstadt, T. H., Newcomb, K., & Funderburk, B. (1991). Parent–child interaction therapy with behavior problem children: Generalization of treatment effects to the school setting. *Journal of Clinical Child Psychology, 20,* 140–151.

McWayne, C., Downer, J. T., Campos, R., & Harris, R. D. (2013). Father involvement during early childhood and its association with children's early learning: A meta-analysis. *Early Education and Development, 24,* 898–922.

MetLife. (2005). *The MetLife survey of the American teacher: Transitions and the role of supportive relationships; A survey of teachers, principals and students.* New York: Author. Retrieved August 4, 2005, from *www.metlife.com/WPSAssets/ 34996838801118758796V1FATS_2004. pdf.*

Mikami, A. Y., Griggs, M. S., Lerner, M. D., Emeh, C. C., Reuland, M. M., Jack, A., et al. (2013). A randomized trial of a classroom intervention to increase peers' social inclusion of children with attention-deficit/hyperactivity disorder. *Journal of Consulting and Clinical Psychology, 81,* 100–112.

Mikami, A. Y., Lerner, M. D., Griggs, M. S., McGrath, A., & Calhoun, C. D. (2010). Parental influences on children with attention-deficit/hyperactivity disorder: II. A pilot intervention training parents as friendship coaches for their children. *Journal of Abnormal Child Psychology, 38*(6), 737–749.

Miller, G. E., & Prinz, R. J. (2003). Engagement of families in treatment for childhood conduct problems. *Behavior Therapy, 34,* 517–534.

Moffitt, T. E. (1993). Adolescence-limited and life-course-persistent antisocial behavior: A developmental taxonomy. *Psychological Review, 100,* 674–701.

Molina, B. S. G., Hinshaw, S. P., Swanson, J. M., Arnold, L. E., Vitiello, B., Jensen, P. S., et al. (2009). MTA at 8 years: Prospective follow-up of children treated for combined type ADHD in a multisite study. *Journal of the American Academy of Child and Adolescent Psychiatry, 48,* 484–500.

Moore Johnson, S., & the Project on the Next Generation of Teachers. (2004). *Finders and keepers: Helping new teachers survive and thrive in our schools.* San Francisco: Jossey-Bass.

MTA Cooperative Group. (1999). A 14-month randomized clinical trial of treatment strategies for attention-deficit/hyperactivity disorder. *Archives of General Psychiatry, 56,* 1073–1086.

National Institute of Mental Health. (2014). Detailed Description of the RDoC Project. Retrieved from *www.nimh.nih.gov/research-priorities/rdoc/index.shtml.*

O'Callaghan, P. M., Reitman, D., Northup, J., Hupp, S. D. A., & Murphy, M. A. (2003). Promoting social skills generalization with ADHD-diagnosed children in a sports setting. *Behavior Therapy, 34,* 313–330.

O'Leary, K. D., Pelham, W. E., Rosenbaum, A., & Price, G. H. (1976). Behavioral treatment of hyperkinetic children. *Clinical Pediatrics, 15,* 510–515.

O'Leary, S. G., & Pelham, W. E. (1978). Behavior therapy and withdrawal of stimulant medication in hyperactive children. *Pediatrics, 61,* 211–217.

Owens, J. S., Goldfine, M. E., Evangelista, N. M., Hoza, B., & Kaiser, N. M. (2007). A critical review of self-perceptions and the positive illusory bias in children with ADHD. *Clinical Child and Family Psychology Review, 10,* 335–351.

Owens, J. S., Murphy, C. E., Richerson, L., Girio, E. L., & Himawan, L. K. (2008). Science to practice in underserved communities: The effectiveness of school mental health programming. *Journal of Clinical Child and Adolescent Psychology, 37,* 434–447.

Page, T. F., Pelham III, W. E., Fabiano, G. A., Greiner, A. R., Gnagy, E. M., Hart, K., et al. (in press). Comparative cost analysis of sequential, adaptive, behavioral, pharmacological, and combined treatments for childhood ADHD. *Journal of Clinical Child and Adolescent Psychology.*

Parke, R. D., McDowell, D. J., Kim, M., Killian, C., Dennis, J., Flyr, M. L., et al. (2002). Fathers' contributions to children's peer relationships. In C. S. Tamis-LeMonda & N. Carbrera (Eds.), *Handbook of father involvement: Interdisciplinary perspectives* (pp. 141–167). Mahwah, NJ: Erlbaum.

Patterson, G. R. (1975a). *Families: Applications of social learning to family life.* Champaign, IL: Research Press.

Patterson, G. R. (1975b). Multiple evaluations of a parent-training program. In J. T. Thompson (Ed.), *Applications of behavior modification* (pp. 299–322). New York: Academic Press.

Patterson, G. R. (1982). *A social learning approach: Vol. 3. Coercive family process.* Eugene, OR: Castalia.

Patterson, G. R., & Forgatch, M. S. (2005). *Parents and adolescents living together: Part 1. The basics* (2nd ed.). Champaign, IL: Research Press.

Patterson, G. R., & Guillon, M. E. (1968). *Living with children: New methods for parents and teachers.* Champaign, IL: Research Press.

Peed, S., Roberts, M., & Forehand, R. (1977). Evaluation of the effectiveness of a standardized parent training program in altering the interaction of mothers and their noncompliant children. *Behavior Modification, 1*, 323–350.

Pelham, W. E. (1993). Pharmacotherapy for children with attention-deficit/hyperactivity disorder. *School Psychology Review, 22*, 199–227.

Pelham, W. E., Burrows-MacLean, L., Gnagy, E. M., Fabiano, G. A., Coles, E., Wymbs, B., et al. (2014). A dose-ranging study of behavioral and pharmacological treatment in social–recreational settings for children with ADHD. *Journal of Abnormal Child Psychology, 42*, 1019–1032.

Pelham, W. E., & Fabiano, G. A. (2008). Evidence-based psychosocial treatment for ADHD: An update. *Journal of Clinical Child and Adolescent Psychology, 37*, 184–214.

Pelham, W. E., Fabiano, G. A., & Massetti, G. M. (2005). Evidence-based assessment for attention-deficit/hyperactivity disorder in children and adolescents. *Journal of Clinical Child and Adolescent Psychology, 34*, 449–476.

Pelham, W. E., Fabiano, G. A., Waxmonsky, J. G., Greiner, A. R., Gnagy, E. M., Pelham III, W. E., et al. (in press). Treatment sequencing for childhood ADHD: A multiple-randomization study of adaptive medication and behavioral interventions. *Journal of Clinical Child and Adolescent Psychology.*

Pelham, W. E., Gnagy, E. M., Burrows-Maclean, L., Williams, A., Fabiano, G. A., Morrissey, S. M., et al. (2001). Once-a-day Concerta™ methylphenidate versus t.i.d. methylphenidate in laboratory and natural settings. *Pediatrics, 107*. Available at *www.pediatrics.org/cgi/content/full/107/6/e105.*

Pelham, W. E., Gnagy, E. M., Chronis, A. M., Burrows-MacLean, L., Fabiano, G. A., Onyango, A. N., et al. (1999). A comparison of morning, midday, and late-afternoon methylphenidate with morning and late-afternoon Adderall in children with attention-deficit/hyperactivity disorder. *Pediatrics, 104*(6), 1300–1311.

Pelham, W. E., Gnagy, E. M., Greenslade, K. E., & Milich, R. (1992). Teacher ratings of DSM-III-R symptoms for the disruptive behavior disorders. *Journal of the American Academy of Child and Adolescent Psychiatry, 31*, 210–218.

Pelham, W. E., Greiner, A. R., & Gnagy, E. M. (1998). *The Children's Summer Treatment Program manual.* Unpublished treatment manual.

Pelham, W. E., Massetti, G. M., Wilson, T., Kipp, H., Myers, D., Newman Standley, B. B., et al. (2005). Implementation of a comprehensive schoolwide behavioral intervention: The ABC Program. *Journal of Attention Disorders, 9*, 248–260.

Pelham, W. E., McBurnett, K., Harper, G. W., Milich, R., Murphy, D. A., Clinton, J., et al. (1990). Methylphenidate and baseball playing in ADHD children: Who's on first? *Journal of Consulting and Clinical Psychology, 58*, 130–133.

Pelham, W. E., Wheeler, T., & Chronis, A. M. (1998). Empirically supported psychosocial treatment for attention deficit hyperactivity disorder. *Journal of Clinical Child Psychology, 27,* 190–205.

Pfiffner, L. J., & McBurnett, K. (1997). Social skills training with parent generalization: Treatment effects for children with attention deficit disorder. *Journal of Consulting and Clinical Psychology, 65,* 749–757.

Pfiffner, L. J., Mikami, A., Huang-Pollock, C., Easterlin, B., Zalecki, C., & McBurnett, K. (2007). A randomized, controlled trial of integrated home–school behavioral treatment for ADHD, predominantly inattentive type. *Journal of the American Academy of Child and Adolescent Psychiatry, 46,* 1041–1050.

Pfiffner, L. J., Villodas, M., Kaiser, N., Rooney, M., & McBurnett, K. (2013). Educational outcomes of a collaborative school–home behavioral intervention for ADHD. *School Psychology Quarterly, 28,* 25–36.

Pinkston, E. M., Reese, N. M., LeBlanc, J. M., & Baer, D. M. (1973). Independent control of a preschool child's aggression and peer interaction by contingent teacher attention. *Journal of Applied Behavior Analysis, 6,* 115–124.

Pisterman, S., Firestone, P., McGrath, P., Goodman, J. T., Webster, I., Mallory, R., et al. (1992). The role of parent training in treatment of preschoolers with ADHD. *American Journal of Orthopsychiatry, 62,* 397–408.

Poulton, A. (2005). Growth on stimulant medication; clarifying the confusion: A review. *Archives of Disease in Childhood, 90,* 801–806.

Power, T. J., Karustis, J. L., & Habboushe, D. F. (2001). *Homework success for children with ADHD: A family–school intervention program.* New York: Guilford Press.

Prinz, R. J., & Miller, G. E. (1994). Family-based treatment for childhood antisocial behavior: Experimental influences on dropout and engagement. *Journal of Consulting and Clinical Psychology, 62,* 645–650.

Prinz, R. J., & Sanders, M. R. (2007). Adopting a population-level approach to parenting and family support interventions. *Clinical Psychology Review, 27,* 739–749.

Reddy, L. A., Fabiano, G. A., Dudek, C. M., & Hsu, L. (2013). Instructional and behavior management practices implemented by elementary general education teachers. *Journal of School Psychology, 51,* 683–700.

Reid, M. J., Webster-Stratton, C., & Hammond, M. (2003). Follow-up of children who received the Incredible Years intervention for oppositional defiant disorder: Maintenance and prediction of 2-year outcome. *Behavior Therapy, 34,* 471–491.

Reid, R., Maag, J. W., Vasa, S. F., & Wright, G. (1994). Who are the children with attention deficit-hyperactivity disorder?: A school-based survey. *Journal of Special Education, 28,* 117–137.

Reyno, S. M., & McGrath, P. J. (2006). Predictors of parent training efficacy for child externalizing behavior problems—a meta-analytic review. *Journal of Child Psychology and Psychiatry, 47,* 99–111.

Roberts, M. W., McMahon, R. J., Forehand, R., & Humphreys, L. (1978). The effect of parental instruction-giving on child compliance. *Behavior Therapy, 9,* 793–798.

Robin, A. L., & Foster, S. L. (1989). *Negotiating parent–adolescent conflict.* New York: Guilford Press.

Robinson, E. A., Eyberg, S. M., & Ross, A. W. (1980). The standardization of an inventory of child conduct problems. *Journal of Clinical Child Psychology, 9,* 22–29.

Rose, L. C., & Gallup, A. M. (2006). The 38th annual Phi Delta Kappa/Gallup Poll of the public's attitudes toward the public schools. *Phi Delta Kappan, 88,* 41–56.

Sanders, M. R. (1999). Triple P-Positive Parenting Program: Towards an empirically validated multilevel parenting and family support strategy for the prevention of behavior and emotional problems in children. *Clinical Child and Family Psychology Review, 2,* 71–90.

Sanders, M. R., Montgomery, D. T., & Brechman-Toussaint, M. L. (2000). The mass media and the prevention of child behavior problems: The evaluation of a television series to promote positive outcome for parents and their children. *Journal of Child Psychology and Psychiatry, 41,* 939–948.

Sanders, M. R., & Turner, K. M. T. (2005). Reflections on the challenges of effective dissemination of behavioural family intervention: Our experience with the Triple P-Positive Parenting Program. *Child and Adolescent Mental Health, 10,* 158–169.

Schlientz, M. D., Riley-Tillman, T. C., Briesch, A. M., Walcott, C. M., & Chafouleas, S. M. (2009). The impact of training on the accuracy of direct behavior ratings (DBR). *School Psychology Quarterly, 24,* 73–83.

Schnoes, C., Reid, R., Wagner, M., & Marder, C. (2006). ADHD among students receiving special education services: A national survey. *Exceptional Children, 72,* 483–496.

Scholer, S. J., Nix, R. L., & Patterson, B. (2006). Gaps in pediatricians' advice to parents regarding early childhood aggression. *Clinical Pediatrics, 45,* 23–28.

Schuhmann, E. M., Foote, R. C., Eyberg, S. M., Boggs, S. R., & Algina, J. (1998). Efficacy of parent–child interaction therapy: Interim report of a randomized trial with short-term maintenance. *Journal of Clinical Child Psychology, 27,* 34–45.

Schultz, B. K., & Evans, S. W. (2015). *A practical guide to implementing school-based interventions for adolescents with ADHD.* New York: Springer.

Schultz, B. K., Evans, S. W., & Serpell, Z. N. (2009). Preventing failure among middle school students with ADHD: A survival analysis. *School Psychology Review, 38,* 14–27.

Scotti, J. R., Morris, T. L., McNeil, C. B., & Hawkins, R. P. (1996). DSM-IV and disorders of childhood and adolescence: Can structural criteria be functional? *Journal of Consulting and Clinical Psychology, 64,* 1177–1191.

Serketich, W. J., & Dumas, J. E. (1996). The effectiveness of behavioral parent training to modify antisocial behavior in children: A meta-analysis. *Behavior Therapy, 27,* 171–186.

Sheridan, S. M., & Kratochwill, T. R. (2008). *Conjoint behavioral consultations: Promoting family-school connections and interventions.* New York: Springer.

Shipstead, Z., Hicks, K. L., & Engle, R. W. (2012). Cogmed working memory training: Does the evidence support the claims? *Journal of Applied Research in Memory and Cognition, 1,* 185–193.

Simmons, D. C., Fuchs, L. S., Fuchs, D., Mathes, P., & Hodge, J. P. (1995). Effects of explicit teaching and peer tutoring on the reading achievement of learning-disabled and low-performing students in regular classrooms. *Elementary School Journal, 95,* 387–408.

Sleator, E. K., Ullmann, R. K., & Von Newmann, A. (1982). How do hyperactive children feel about taking stimulants and will they tell the doctor? *Clinical Pediatrics, 21,* 474–479.

Sonuga-Barke, E. J. S., Brandeis, D., Cortese, S., Daley, D., Ferrin, M., Holtmann, M., et al. (2013). Nonpharmalogical interventions for ADHD: Systematic review and meta-analyses of randomized controlled trials of dietary and psychological treatments. *American Journal of Psychiatry, 170,* 275–289.

Sonuga-Barke, E. J. S., Daley, D., & Thompson, M. (2002). Does maternal ADHD reduce the effectiveness of parent training for preschool children's ADHD? *Journal of the American Academy of Child and Adolescent Psychiatry, 41,* 696–702.

Steege, M. W., & Watson, T. S. (2009). *Conducting school-based functional behavioral assessments: A practitioner's guide* (2nd ed.). New York: Guilford Press.

Stichter, J. P., Lewis, T. J., Whittaker, T. A., Richter, M., Johnson, N. W., & Trussell, R. P. (2009). Assessing teacher use of opportunities to respond and effective classroom management strategies: Comparisons among high- and low-risk elementary schools. *Journal of Positive Behavioral Interventions, 11,* 68–81.

Stokes, T. F., & Baer, D. M. (1977). An implicit technology of generalization. *Journal of Applied Behavior Analysis, 10,* 349–367.

Stormont-Spurgin, M., & Zentall, S. (2006). Child-rearing practices associated with aggression in youth with and without ADHD: An exploratory study. *International Journal of Disability, 43,* 135–146.

Stormshak, E. A., & Dishion, T. J. (2002). An ecological approach to child and family clinical and counseling psychology. *Clinical Child and Family Psychology Review, 5,* 197–215.

Sugai, G., & Colvin, G. (1997). Debriefing: A transition step for promoting acceptable behavior. *Education and Treatment of Children, 20,* 209–221.

Sugai, G., Horner, R. H., Dunlap, G., Hieneman, M., Lewis, T. J., Nelson, C. M., et al. (1999). *Applying positive behavioral support and functional behavioral assessment in schools. Technical assistance guide 1, Version 1.4.3.* Washington, DC: Center on Positive Behavioral Interventions and Support (OSEP).

Sutherland, K. S., & Wehby, J. H. (2001). Exploring the relationship between increased opportunities to respond to academic requests and the academic and behavioral outcomes of students with EBD: A review. *Remedial and Special Education, 22,* 113–121.

Swanson, J. M., Elliott, G. R., Greenhill, L. L., Wigal, T., Arnold, L. E., Vitiello, B., et al. (2007). Effects of stimulant medication on growth rates across 3 years in the MTA follow-up. *Journal of the American Academy of Child and Adolescent Psychiatry, 46,* 1015–1027.

Todd, A. W., Campbell, A. L., Meyer, G. G., & Horner, R. H. (2008). The effects of a targeted intervention to reduce problem behaviors: Elementary school implementation of Check In–Check Out. *Journal of Positive Behavior Interventions, 10,* 46–55.

U.S. Food and Drug Administration. (2011). FDA drug safety communication: Safety review update of medications used to treat attention-deficit/hyperactivity disorder (ADHD) in children and young adults. Retrieved from *www.fda.gov/Drugs/DrugSafety/ucm277770.htm.*

Vannest, K. J., Davis, J. L., Davis, C. R., Mason, B. A., & Burke, M. D. (2010). Effective intervention for behavior with a daily behavior report card: A meta-analysis. *School Psychology Review, 39,* 654–672.

Visser, S. N., & Lesesne, C. A. (2005). Mental health in the United States: Prevalence of diagnosis and medication treatment for attention-deficit/hyperactivity disorder—United States, 2003. *Morbidity and Mortality Weekly Report, 54,* 842–847.

Volpe, R., & Fabiano, G. A. (2013). *Daily behavior report cards: An evidence-based system of assessment and intervention.* New York: Guilford Press.

Vujnovic, R. K., Fabiano, G. A., Morris, K., Norman, K. E., Hallmark, C., & Hartley, C. (2014). Examining school psychologists' and teachers' application of approaches within a response to intervention (RTI) framework. *Exceptionality, 22*(3), 129–140.

Walker, H. M. (2015). Perspectives on seminal achievements and challenges in the field of emotional and behavioral disorders. *Remedial and Special Education, 36,* 39–44.

Walker, H. M., Colvin, G., & Ramsey, E. (1994). *Antisocial behavior in school: Strategies and best practices.* New York: Wadsworth.

Walker, H. M., & Eaton-Walker, J. (1991). *Coping with noncompliance in the classroom.* Austin, TX: PRO-ED.

Walker, H. M., Ramsey, E., & Gresham, F. M. (2003). *Antisocial behavior in schools: Evidence-based practices.* New York: Cengage Learning.

Walker, H. M., Severson, H., & Feil, E. (2014). *Systematic screening for behavior disorders* (2nd ed.). Eugene, OR: Pacific Northwest.

Walker, H. M., Severson, H., Seeley, J., Feil, E., Small, J., Golly, A., et al. (2014). The evidence base of the First Step to Success early intervention for preventing emerging antisocial behavior patterns. In H. M. Walker & F. M. Gresham (Eds.), *Handbook of evidence-based practices for emotional and behavioral disorders: Applications in schools* (pp. 518–534). New York: Guilford Press.

Waschbusch, D. A., Cunningham, C. E., Pelham, W. E., Rimas, H. L., Greiner, A. R., Gnagy, E. M., et al. (2011). A discrete choice conjoint experiment to evaluate parent preferences for treatment of young, medication naïve children with ADHD. *Journal of Clinical Child and Adolescent Psychology, 40,* 546–561.

Webster-Stratton, C. (1997). *The incredible years: A trouble-shooting guide for parents of children aged 3–8.* Toronto: Umbrella Press.

Webster-Stratton, C. (2005). The incredible years: A training series for the prevention and treatment of conduct problems in young children. In E. D. Hibbs & P. S. Jensen (Eds.), *Psychosocial treatments for child and adolescent disorders* (2nd ed., pp. 507–555). Washington, DC: American Psychological Association.

Webster-Stratton, C., Reid, J. M., & Hammond, M. (2004). Treating children with early-onset conduct problems: Intervention outcome for parent, child, and teacher training. *Journal of Clinical Child and Adolescent Psychology, 33,* 105–124.

Webster-Stratton, C., Reid, J. M., & Stoolmiller, M. (2008). Preventing conduct problems and improving school readiness: Evaluation of the Incredible Years Teacher and Child Training Programs in high-risk schools. *Journal of Child Psychology and Psychiatry and Allied Disciplines, 49,* 471–488.

Wells, K. C., Chi, T. C., Hinshaw, S. P., Epstein, J. N., Pfiffner, L. J., Nebel-Schwain, M., et al. (2006). Treatment-related changes in objectively measured parenting behaviors in the multimodal treatment study of children with ADHD. *Journal of Consulting and Clinical Psychology, 74,* 649–657.

Wells, K. C., Pelham, W. E., Kotkin, R. A., Hoza, B., Abikoff, H. B., Abramowitz, A., et al. (2000). Psychosocial treatment strategies in the MTA study: Rationale, methods, and critical issues in the design and implementation. *Journal of Abnormal Child Psychology, 28,* 483–505.

White, M. A. (1975). Natural rates of teacher approval and disapproval in the classroom. *Journal of Applied Behavioral Analysis, 8,* 367–372.

Witt, J. C., & Elliott, S. N. (1982). The response cost lottery: A time efficient and effective classroom intervention. *Journal of School Psychology, 20,* 155–161.

Wolraich, M. L., Wilson, D. B., & White, J. W. (1995). The effects of sugar on behavior or cognition in children: A meta-analysis. *Journal of the American Medical Association, 274,* 1617–1621.

Zentall, S. S., & Goldstein, S. (1999). *Seven steps to homework success: A family guide for solving common homework problems.* Plantation, FL: Specialty Press.

Zuvekas, S. H., Vitiello, B., & Norquist, G. S. (2006). Recent trends in stimulant medication use among U.S. children. *American Journal of Psychiatry, 163,* 579–585.

Index

Page numbers followed by *f* indicate figure, *t* indicate table